SOCIAL JUSTICE IN CLINICAL PRACTICE

Social work theory and ethics place social justice at the core of social work practice. However, social justice work has all too often been conceptualized as a macro intervention, separate and distinct from clinical practice.

This practical text is designed to help social workers to intervene around the impact of socio-political factors with their clients and to integrate social justice into their clinical work. Based on past radical traditions, it introduces and applies a liberation health framework which merges clinical and macro work into a singular, unified way of working with individuals, families and communities. Opening with a chapter on the theory and historical roots of liberation social work practice, each subsequent chapter goes on to look at a particular population group or individual case study, including:

- LGBT communities
- mental health
- violence
- addiction
- cultural groups
- housing issues.

Written by a team of experienced lecturers and practitioners, *Social Justice in Clinical Practice* provides a clear, focused, practice-oriented model of clinical social work for both social work practitioners and students.

Dawn Belkin Martinez is Lecturer in Clinical Practice at the Boston University School of Social Work, USA, and formerly an instructor in psychiatry at Harvard Medical School. She is one of the founding members of the Boston Liberation Health Group and gives presentations locally, nationally and internationally about her work with immigrant families, liberation health theory and practice, and social justice.

Ann Fleck-Henderson is Professor Emerita at Simmons College School of Social Work, USA, and a consultant on intimate violence issues and on social work curriculum and pedagogy.

SOCIAL JUSTICE IN CLINICAL PRACTICE

A liberation health framework for social work

Edited by Dawn Belkin Martinez and Ann Fleck-Henderson

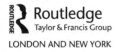

Routledge
Taylor & Francis Group

LONDON AND NEW YORK

First published 2014
by Routledge
2 Park Square, Milton Park, Abingdon, Oxon, OX14 4RN

and by Routledge
711 Third Avenue, New York, NY 10017
Routledge is an imprint of the Taylor and Francis Group, an informa business

The editors would like to acknowledge Paul Saba for his editorial and intellectual
support and Simmons College for its financial contributions to the book.

British Library Cataloguing in Publication Data
A catalogue record for this book is available from the British Library

Library of Congress Cataloging in Publication Data
Social justice in clinical practice : a liberation health framework for social work /
edited by Dawn Belkin Martinez and Ann Fleck-Henderson.
pages cm

1. Social service--Moral and ethical aspects. 2. Social justice. I. Martinez, Dawn
Belkin. II. Fleck-Henderson, Ann.
HV10.5.S615 2014
362.1'0425--dc23
2013035562

ISBN: 978-0-415-69895-5 (hbk)
ISBN: 978-0-415-69896-2 (pbk)
ISBN: 978-1-315-81307-3 (ebk)

Typeset in Bembo
by FiSH Books, London

CONTENTS

LIST OF FIGURES

CONTRIBUTORS

Jackie Savage Borne Clinical social worker, advocate and program manager at a hospital-based domestic violence intervention program, Cambridge, MA.

Liana Buccieri Clinical social worker, Boston University Student Health Services, Boston, MA.

Ezekiel Reis Burgin Social worker in community practice.

Estela Pérez Bustillo Social worker in community practice, Boston, MA.

Ann Fleck-Henderson PhD, Professor Emerita, Simmons College School of Social Work, Cambridge, MA.

Chloe Frankel Social services advocate, Committee for Public Counsel Services, Somerville, MA.

Johnnie Hamilton-Mason PhD, Professor, Simmons College School of Social Work, Hyde Park, MA.

Jared Douglas Kant Social worker in community practice.

Dawn Belkin Martinez PhD, Lecturer in Clinical Practice, Boston University School of Social Work, Boston, MA. Clinical social worker, Boston University Student Health Services, Wellness and Prevention Services.

Eleana McMurry Emergency Services Clinician, North Suffolk Mental Health Association, Boston, MA.

Zack Osheroff Program Manager and Therapeutic Mentor, Friends of the Children-Boston, Boston, MA.

Carol Swenson PhD, Professor Emerita, Simmons College School of Social Work, Boston, MA.

Anne Vinick Community social worker in lower-income housing communities.

INTRODUCTION

Why liberation health social work?

Dawn Belkin Martinez

The world in crisis

Over the past 30 years, the United States, like the rest of the developed world, has witnessed a fundamental transformation of its economy and society under the impact of rampant neo-liberalism.[1] The results have been a growth of inequality, poverty and social dislocation, a significant privatization of public services, and the messaging of an ideology that privileges the market above community and personal advancement above social welfare (Ferguson and Lavalette 2013). A brief review of statistics from the United States presents a devastating picture.

Growth of inequality

Today, the top one percent of all US households earns seventy times as much as the bottom 20 percent of households. This difference is more than three times what it was 30 years ago (Reisch 2013; Sherman and Stone 2010). In the United States, the share of national assets owned by the richest one percent of households has grown from one-fifth to over one-third of all private wealth; this represents the most unequal distribution of the nation's wealth since 1928, the beginning of the great depression (Reisch, 2013).

Increase in poverty

In his article "What is the Future of Social Work?" Michael Reisch reports that there are now 50 million people who are officially poor, "the largest number of people living in poverty since the US began to measure poverty" (Reisch 2013:71; US Census Bureau 2012). Monea and Sawhill (2010) claim that if the official poverty line was adjusted to account for increases in acceptable living standards, about one-third of the nation's population (100 million people) would be considered poor. Currently, approximately one-quarter of all African-Americans and Latinos are living in poverty (Buss 2010).

Crisis in the housing

Home foreclosures have increased nine percent since 2011–12. While is difficult to obtain specific statistics regarding the number of homeless individuals, it is estimated that there are at least 630,000 people on any given evening that are considered homeless. These figures do not include an estimated 6.8 million who are currently doubled up with friends and families (National Alliance to End Homelessness 2013).

An increase in food insecurity

According to the US Department of Agriculture, there are currently 50 million people in the United States, one of every six Americans, who experience food insufficiency (Reisch 2013; US Department of Agriculture 2012).

Growing incarceration rates

Today, there are more African-Americans who are under the control of the criminal justice system (prison/jail, probation/parole) than were enslaved in 1850. In 2001 one in six African-American men were incarcerated, and the number is increasing. If current trends continue, one in three African-American males born today can expect to spend time in prison during his lifetime (Alexander 2010; NAACP 2013).

The crisis and mainstream social work practice

Needless to say, neo-liberalism's impact on the social-work profession has been ongoing and dramatic. Many social workers find themselves overwhelmed by the number of clients they are required to see, at the same time that they face reduced resources and limited options in the way of services they can provide. The shredding of the social safety net, a hallmark of the former New Deal welfare system, has dramatically altered the institutional context in which much social work occurs, while the new neo-liberal consensus has imposed new legal, institutional and organizational constraints on social work practice, public and private.

To date, social work has had difficulty fashioning an adequate response to these developments. Perhaps most tragically, neo-liberalism has undermined social work's long-standing ethical foundations, compelling social workers to increasingly focus their practice with clients and communities according to the logic of the market and the financial "bottom line." This approach stands in stark contrast to the stated ethical goals which have been central to the social work narrative since its emergence as a profession.

The ethical imperatives of social work have always included a specific commitment to social and economic justice and to individual and collective empowerment (Reisch 2013). While at times over the years, these commitments were honored more in theory than in practice, they still have exercised a powerful influence, particularly among social workers just coming into the profession and those who found their calling in the 1930s, late 1960s, and early 1970s.

Neo-liberalism, in theory and practice, is fundamentally antithetical to social work's ethical foundations. Its ideological assumptions run counter to what the best of traditional social work taught. It promotes individualism – the belief that individuals are fundamentally on their own. It argues that whether an individual sinks or swims is up to that individual. Society, much less the government, has no obligation to lend a helping hand. It insists that the "invisible hand" of the market, if left alone to do its work, will provide benefits for all who conform to its norms.

This ideology has had a corrosive impact on social work theory, influencing practitioners' values, beliefs, assumptions and attitudes. And it has had an equally harmful impact on the profession's practice, compelling clinical social workers to increasingly devote their attention to assisting clients to adapt their thinking and behavior to the "new normal" of the neo-liberal social order rather than working with them to challenge it.

The combination of increased social dysfunction resulting from implementation of the neo-liberal agenda in society at large and the challenges of the mainstream social work response have resulted in a growing crisis in the profession and the proliferation of opportunities for alternative theories and approaches in social work to gain a hearing.

Liberation health social work

Previous generations of social workers, particularly during the Great Depression, and again starting in the 1960s, worked in periods of deep social crisis similar to the present, and the challenges of their times moved them to call into question many of social work's dominant paradigms. They pointed to inadequacies in mainstream social-work models and struggled to develop effective alternatives (Brake and Bailey 1980; Corrigan and Leonard 1978; Ferguson 2009; Fook 1993; Lavalette 2011; Lee 1994; Reisch and Andrews 2002; Specht and Coutney 1994.) Their critiques targeted in particular the profession's focus on individualizing social problems and, as a consequence, developing individualized solutions, while minimizing the structural and institutional factors contributing to clients' problems (Reisch 2013). They looked to a range of social movements outside the social work field to ally with in a common fight for a more just and equal world. These social workers forged a rich radical tradition, the memory of which has largely been forgotten today.

The liberation health social work model is a product of the current social, economic, and political crisis. Believing that "another social work is possible!"

(Ferguson 2009), it builds on past radical traditions while seeking to develop new paradigms for social work appropriate for our current crisis. It shares this goal with a significant number of social workers around the world who are also looking for critical and radical ideas to help explain the problems social workers and clients experience and offers a guide to an alternative social work practice (Ferguson and Lavalette 2013).

The liberation health social-work model seeks to provide practitioners with practical tools for effective clinical work in the era of neo-liberalism. Embedded in these practical tools, however, are broader visions of what social work should be. Liberation health envisions a practice of social work that is:

- holistic: situating individuals' problems in their full matrix of personal, structural, institutional and ideological determinants;
- critical: refusing to accept neo-liberalism and refusing to accept the notion that social work ought to subordinate itself to its social agenda;
- empowering: seeking to liberate clients and social workers from the confining belief that current conditions are inevitable and beyond our power to change; seeking to support their becoming active allies of individuals and movements working for social change;
- hopeful: rescuing the memory of and valuing "the collective human capacity to create change" (Reisch 2013: 68).

Finally, it is important to note that the vast majority of clinical situations presented in this book can be considered "success stories"; that is, the client or family member found the work to be helpful. As with all practice theories, there are many examples of clients not finding the work to be helpful. For the purposes of this book, we deliberately chose examples which would help us to teach this theory of practice and to offer hope that another model of clinical social work is possible. In every case, we hope that our asking the kinds of questions described in this book plants a seed for both clients and social workers to think about clinical issues differently; to see themselves and their problems as part of a much larger sociopolitical system and to take action, in whatever way they feel will be helpful. To paraphrase Reisch and Andrews (2002), the road to liberation practice might be the road not taken, but this road not taken lies ahead (p. 235).

Note

1   Neo-liberalism is a form of capitalism, developed at the end of the 20th century, which seeks to radically restructure society by dismantling social welfare systems and promoting policies that increasingly shift social wealth and political power to corporations and the rich at the expense of the majority of the population. See also George (1999).

References

Alexander, M. (2010) *The New Jim Crow: Mass Incarceration in the Age of Colorblindness*. New York: New Press.

Brake, M. and Bailey, R. (eds) (1980) *Radical Social Work and Practice*. London: Edward Arnold.

Buss, J. A. (2010) Have the poor gotten poorer? The American experience from 1987–2007. *Journal of Poverty*, 14 (2): 93–107.

Corrigan, P. and Leonard, P. (1978) *Social Work Practice Under Capitalism: A Marxist Approach*. London: Macmillian.

Ferguson, I. (2009) Another social work is possible: Reclaiming the radical tradition. In V. Leskosek (ed.), *Theories and Methods of Social Work: Exploring Different Perspectives*. Ljubljana, Slovenia: Faculty of Social Work, University of Ljubljana, pp. 81–98.

Ferguson, I. and Lavalette, M. (2013) Critical and radical social work: An introduction. *Critical and Radical Social Work*, 1 (1): 3–14.

Fook, J. (1993) *Radical Casework: A Theory of Practice*. St. Leonards, NSW: Allen and Unwin.

George, S. (1999) A short history of neoliberalism: Twenty years of elite economics and emerging opportunities for structural change. Conference on Economic Sovereignty in a Globalising World, Bangkok, 24–26 March 1999. Global Exchange. Available online at www.globalexchange.org/resources/econ101/neoliberalismhist (accessed October 1, 2013).

Lavalette, M. (2011) *Radical Social Work Today: Social Work at the Crossroads*. Bristol: Policy Press.

Lee, J. (1994) *The Empowerment Approach to Social Work Practice*. New York: Columbia University Press.

Monea, E. and Sawhill, I. (2010) *A Simulation on Future Poverty in the United States*. Washington DC: Urban Institute.

NAACP (2013) National Association for the Advancement of Colored People, Criminal Justice Fact Sheet. Available online at www.naacp.org/pages/criminal-justice-fact-sheet (accessed October 1, 2013).

National Alliance to End Homelessness, Homelessness Research Institute (2013) *State of Homelessness in America 2013*. Washington, DC: National Alliance to End Homelessness. Available online at www.endhomelessness.org/library/entry/the-state-of-homelessness-2013 (accessed October 1, 2013).

Reisch, M. (2013) What is the future of social work? *Critical and Radical Social Work* 1(1): 67–85.

Reisch, M. and Andrews, J. (2002) *The Road Not Taken: A History of Radical Social Work in the United States*. London: Brunner-Routledge.

Sherman, A. and Stone, C. (2010) Income gaps between very rich and everyone else more than tripled in the last three decades, new data show. Center on Budget and Policy Priorities. Available online at www.cbpp.org/cms/?fa=viewandid=3220 (accessed October 1, 2013).

Specht, H. and Courtney, M. (1994) *Unfaithful Angels: How Social Work Abandoned its Mission*. New York: Free Press.

US Census Bureau (2012) *Statistics on Poverty in the United States*. Washington, DC: US Government Printing Office.

US Department of Agriculture (2012) Statistics on the Supplemental Nutritional Assistance Program. Washington, DC: US Government Printing Office.

OVERVIEW OF THE BOOK

Ann Fleck-Henderson

This book consists of chapters by different authors, each of whom is involved in the liberation health movement and is a member of the liberation health group in Boston, Massachusetts. Each of the authors describes clinical social work done from a liberation health perspective in a social work agency. Many of the authors have recently received their masters degrees in social work, and you will notice that some of the chapters describe work done while the writer was an intern. The group of writers met monthly over a couple of years to discuss each chapter as it was being written. This collective and collaborative process is consistent with the approach of liberation health.

As you can see from the table of contents, the book begins with a chapter by Dawn Belkin Martinez, which presents the theory of liberation social-work practice. This includes a summary of its historical roots in education, psychology and social work, and an outline of its essential philosophical, moral and theoretical components. In the second chapter, Jared Kant describes his experience of becoming a liberation health social worker as a masters in social work student. These two chapters should be read first. Each of the subsequent chapters is identified by a population group or an issue. They can be read in any order, and it makes sense to follow your own interests.

Starting with Chapter 2, each chapter has a similar format: introduction to the setting, literature review, case presentation and reflection. You will see that the authors vary in style and even in political perspective. We hope those differences will be thought-provoking to readers, and that the common organization and use of the same visual tool to organize the formulations will help provide coherence across chapters.

The case presentation is the heart of each of these chapters. The first part of that section contains identifying information, referral and presenting concerns, current situation and relevant history. A liberation health formulation follows, and then description of interventions. Each chapter also includes a visual "triangle" illustrating the author's formulation. In order to fully protect the privacy of real clients, each of these cases is significantly disguised. Either the case is a composite of a number of real people; or, in a few chapters, the client has collaborated in producing the narrative, which is still disguised.

Each chapter focuses, particularly in the literature review, on the group or issue for which it is named. The work described also centers on that identity or issue. This seems a useful device for organizing the book and conveying both knowledge and a practice example. Nonetheless, in every case, the particular person with whom the author is working has multiple identities and varied concerns and issues. In order to condense the work done and to maintain the focus on an issue or identity, the authors necessarily omitted some of the complexity. No person is adequately described by a population group or an issue; each of the people you will meet in these chapters is as complex as you or me.

In Chapter 3, Ezekiel Bergin speaks about work with sexual and gender minorities, raising important questions about pronouns and about different challenges for clinicians who are or are not also gender/sexual minorities. The client presented, a young Asian-American man who identifies as male, although born female, dramatically illustrates the relation of dominant world-view assumptions to psychological pain.

Major mental illness in the community is the subject of Chloe Frankel's chapter (Chapter 4). Her client becomes homeless, a high risk for those dealing with serious mental illness. The work involves examining roots of her stereotypes about mental illness and homelessness, and then making new connections and beginning more active self-advocacy.

A dedicated domestic violence service in a large urban hospital is the setting for work described in the chapter by Ann Fleck-Henderson and Jacqueline Savage Borne (Chapter 5). The client, an immigrant woman of color, had been abused for many years by her husband. This chapter draws on literature of the battered women's movement and feminist psychology, as well as liberation health. The case discussion illustrates the importance of support and solidarity with others facing similar challenges.

Liana Buccieri's chapter (Chapter 6) presents work in an outpatient addiction treatment program, beginning with a review of varied practice approaches to this work. Her interventions involve drawing attention to the unexamined assumptions that underlie much of the male client's worldview, many related to cultural and class norms about gender, emotion and independence. The client's becoming reflective about those assumptions changes their role in his behavior.

Johnnie Hamilton-Mason's chapter on work with African-Americans underscores the importance of the common history of colonization and oppression for people of African descent in the Americas. It is important to the work that both client and clinician share this history. Themes of historical legacy, family resilience, cultural gender prescriptions and the importance of the black church are central to their analysis.

Although we do not think of privileged and upper-middle-class people as oppressed, they too are burdened with cultural assumptions and expectations which can contribute to psychological pain. Eleana McMurray's chapter (Chapter 7) illustrates the ways in which aspects of our economy and our culture can be harmful even for those who seem to be "the winners."

Child welfare work is particularly challenging for liberation health social workers because of the power that the social worker holds as an agent of the State. The chapter by Zack Osheroff (Chapter 9) references some of the particular dilemmas in this work. He describes a colleague's intervention in her public child welfare office to address the problem of negative talk about clients.

Anne Vinick's chapter, written with Carol Swenson, describes work in a public housing community (Chapter 10). The defined community, where residents share common concerns, has advantages for liberation work. The social worker is part of the immediate community and of an institution central to the client's life. At the same time, as Anne indicates, her position as both a management employee and an advocate for residents' needs has intrinsic tension.

Chapter 11 presents work on an inpatient psychiatric unit with an adolescent and her family. The chapter illustrates the ways in which each of the family members moves beyond seeing the problem only as the behavior of the hospitalized teen. Dawn Belkin Martinez points out how her approach is similar to other family therapy practice, but differs in its explicit attention to the linkages between personal pain and public issues/cultural norms. This chapter also shows how the clinical team on the unit was involved with the treatment.

The final chapter, by Estela Perez Bastillo, describes work with an adolescent from El Salvador who has reunited with his mother after an eight-year separation, during which he lived with relatives in his home country, while she worked in the United States to support the family. As a newly arrived undocumented immigrant, the client has struggles with his mother, drops out of school, is depressed and impulsive. The chapter describes his beginning to see his situation in a larger context, while he also is helped to find new resources.

The purpose of the book is to introduce clinical social workers to a way of working that fully attends to the cultural and institutional sources of personal troubles, as well as the biopsychological and familial ones. This approach begins with keen observation of and attention to the person or people one hopes to help. Listening well, conveying empathy, understanding the concerns of the other is the foundation of this work, as it is of all clinical work. If we do not emphasize those skills in this book, it is only because we assume that they are being learned and practiced already.

The book suggests a method of analysis and directions for interventions. However, it would not be liberating work if it became a simple application of techniques. Liberation formulations and interventions must be rooted in and follow the clients' own concerns and hopes. Insofar as they introduce new information and new ways of thinking to the person one hopes to help, those must be held and offered with humility and with respect for the fact that, in the end, you are an outsider to the other's experience.

1

THE LIBERATION HEALTH MODEL

Theory and practice

Dawn Belkin Martinez

Introduction

In this chapter, we cover the principal theoretical and practical sources of the liberation health social work model and provide an overview of general liberation health social work methods and practices with an emphasis on clinical work. We end with a brief summary of liberation health and related radical social work resources.

Sources of liberation health theory

Liberation health theory draws from three different conceptual frameworks and practices: Paulo Freire and popular education, liberation psychology, and the radical social work tradition in the United States.

Paulo Freire and popular education

Paulo Freire was a Brazilian educator and theorist best known for his book, *Pedagogy of the Oppressed* (1998). In the 1950s, Freire initiated a national literacy program, supported by the Catholic Church and a number of community organizations in the Brazilian state of Pernambuco for the urban and rural poor. In developing the program, Freire was particularly influenced by a grassroots organization called Catholic Action, a coalition of university students and workers teaching low-income, illiterate community members to read, write and organize themselves in order to play a more active role in Brazilian society. During their meetings, Catholic Action members would discuss ongoing problems, seek to identify their roots causes, and develop action plans to address identified problems (Castano, Castano, and Paulo 1993; Freire 1974).

Freire began working with Catholic Action to help them expand the literacy campaign. Through their efforts in the field, they discovered that many of the individuals with whom they were working shared a fatalistic attitude toward their lives, believing that it was impossible to change their individual circumstances and resigning themselves to their situation or "fate" in society (Castano, Castano, and Paulo 1993). As a result, Freire and Catholic Action decided to use the literacy campaign to do more than just encourage reading and writing; they wanted to challenge and help transform the social consciousness of Brazilian workers.

To do so, Freire and his colleagues further developed the Catholic Action method of seeking to identify the problems that workers were experiencing, to analyze the root causes of these problems, and then to act to change the situation. They soon discovered that when workers started to talk, analyze and act on the problems in their communities, they began to free themselves from their fatalism, challenging both internal voices of passivity and the negative messages they had received from society about themselves (Freire 1974). This new method of promoting literacy and empowerment was enormously successful. After Freire and his colleagues were able to teach 300 illiterate sugarcane workers to read in just 45 days, the Brazilian government decided to replicate the model, sponsoring thousands of "cultural circles," programs for the development of literacy and critical consciousness. Through his work with these cultural learning circles, Freire further developed his conceptual framework and methods, which are known today as "popular education" (Freire 1974; Torres and Fischman 1994).

Popular education seeks to mobilize and organize people, with the goal of creating popular power (Freire 1974). Many of the components of Paulo Freire's framework are extremely relevant for liberation health theory and practice, with the concept of "knowledge" being seminal. For Freire and his colleagues, the concept of "knowledge" is an historically determined social construct. Both knowledge and the methods used to teach it are not neutral; on the contrary, they are the product of specific historical moments and reflect the ideas and beliefs (worldview) of definite social groups.

In general, the dominant modes of education in a society largely reflect and teach the worldview of the dominant class. The people who exercise social power define what "knowledge" is, and that "knowledge" serves to promote their interests and reinforce their power. Freire believed that what students are traditionally taught and how they are traditionally taught it under capitalism (what he called the banking concept of education) served the political agenda of the capitalist class (Bartlett 2005; Freire 1970).

Freire proposed a completely different framework for education, starting from his distinction between individuals as "objects and subjects" (Freire 1970, 1974). Freire distinguished between an object-like experience and a subject-like experience of life. "Subjects" were people who believed they could act upon the world; they generally had high levels of self-efficacy, causal importance and positive self-concepts. Subjects not only had critical skills for influencing the institutions that exercised control over their lives, they also sought out opportunities to exercise these skills (Freire 1996, 1998).

Objects were people whose experience of life was one of being acted on by others. The less control that individuals believe they have over their lives, the less confidence they have in their ability or likelihood of changing them, the more these individuals will experience the world as "acting on" them. For Freire and his colleagues, the kinds of knowledge people received and the ways they were taught it were major influences on their self perception as subjects or objects (Freire, 1970, 1974, 1996, 1998).

Drawing on his experience with Catholic Action, Freire put forth the idea that students as much as teachers need to be the subjects of the learning process, just as they needed to be the *subjects* of their own destinies. Moreover, students and educators need to be equal participants in the learning process. In this way, the educational process develops as a continuous dialogue between educators and learners. Freire argued that the goal of education is to liberate the learners/students from their external and internal oppression and to render them capable of changing their lives and their societies. Through ongoing open dialogue about their lives, through posing problems and challenging themselves to develop solutions, students develop a critical consciousness of themselves and their world. This educational method Freire called "reading the world" (Belkin Martinez 2004; Castano, Castano, and Paulo 1993).

"Freedom or Liberation is acquired by conquest, it is not a gift … it must be pursued constantly and responsibly." "'Conscientization' or critical consciousness … is daring to perceive social, political, and economic contradictions and to take action against the oppressive elements of reality" (Freire 1970: 35).

Methods and practice of popular education

Although Freire was not a social worker, he has had a significant influence on social work practice. In her article "Paulo Freire, Neglected Mentor for Social Work," Rebecca Hegar reports that a review of the literature (social work abstracts and social science citation index) yields more than 300 articles about Freire, including 18 articles directly related to social work practice (Heger 2012). Some of the topics discussed in these articles include the implications of Freire's work for social work practice with the homeless community (Kline, Dolgon, and Dresser 2000), in the healthcare field, (Aambo 1997) and for developing empowerment-oriented practice (Breton 1994).

This influence on social-work practice is particularly remarkable given the highly theoretical nature of much of Paulo Freire's writings; some critics have charged that his ideas are devoid of practical applications and specific techniques (Belkin Martinez 2004; Castano, Castano and Paulo 1993). Freire was reluctant to develop a specific methodology. He believed that each practical experience with each group of learners was different and that the role of educators was to develop their own activities and techniques with the people with whom they were working. However, he did employ a "method" for facilitating dialogue and consciousness raising. While he was not the only one writing about these methods, he is the educator most closely associated with the popular education movement. (Torres and Fischman 1994).

Among the most important elements of the practice of popular education that have influenced the development of the liberation health social work model are the following:

- First, an individual's lived experience and more importantly, the collective experience of a group (previous experience or previous knowledge) is the beginning basis for their "education" process. Freireian work emphasizes the shared experiences of the learners/subjects as a group rather than privileging the individual experience (Freire 1974, 1998).
- Second, although Freire was critical of developing specific methods to practice, most Freireian educational processes includes three basic steps: (1) seeing a problem as experienced by learners; (2) analyzing the root causes of the problem; (3) developing an action plan to address the problem.
- Third, "reading the world" involves learners reflecting critically on their experiences and knowledge; in order to challenge taken-for-granted assumptions and myths about the world, to "demystify existing forms of false consciousness" (Torres and Fischman 1994: 82).

Liberation psychology

Ignacio Martín-Baró, a Latino social psychologist and Jesuit priest who was born in Spain but spent most of his adult life in El Salvador, is considered the father of liberation psychology (Burton and Kegan 2005). Starting in Latin America, the liberation psychology movement later spread to Europe and North America. In particular, it found important adherents in Ireland, with its complex history of colonial and post colonial legacies (hooks 1993; Fanon 1967; Moane 2010).

Martín-Baró was critical of traditional theories of psychology and what he saw as their limited view of the causes of psychological problems. In particular, he believed that these theories failed to recognize and address the nexus between psychological problems and structural injustice. Familiar with the theories and practice of liberation theology, he sought to apply its insights to the creation of a new psychology. In his most famous work, *Writings for a Liberation Psychology*, Martín-Baró rejected the idea of an impartial, objective psychology and wrote that the root causes of oppression lie in structures, political, economic, cultural, and the worldviews that underlie and reinforce oppressive social conditions (Martín-Baró 1994). The effects of these structures and worldviews are internalized by subordinate groups (internalized oppression) and reinforce their lived experiences of deprivation, violence, poverty, and stress.

The goal of liberation psychology, like Freire's popular education movement, is to transform both the individual and society (Martín-Baró 1994). Martín-Baró described this process as the "breaking of chains of personal oppression as much as the chains of social oppression" (Martín-Baró 1994: 27). In her review of liberation psychology literature, Geraldine Moane, an Irish psychologist, notes the similarities between liberation psychology, feminist psychology, and the community psychology movement; all three theories of practice focus on oppressive socio-political conditions as major factors which contribute to psychological problems and all three emphasize empowerment and personal/social transformation as the goals of intervention (Moane 2003).

Building on Freire's understanding of the historical connection between personal problems and dominant worldview messaging, Martín-Baró called for a liberation psychology which would be focused on de-ideologizing' knowledge and taken for granted assumptions. Like Freire, he emphasized the importance of "critical consciousness." Liberation psychology would help people to understand how their personal problems were directly connected to the institutions and social practices of the societies in which they lived and to the ideologies associated with them (ideas around race, class, gender, consumerism, individualism, competition, and sexual preference, for example) (Belkin Martinez 2004; Burton and Kegan 2005; Martín-Baró 1994; Montero and Sonn 2009).

Moane argues that understanding how oppressive messages become internalized into an individual's personality or psyche is a crucial element in the connection between social conditions of oppression (racism, classism, sexism etc.) and psychological patterns of oppression.

"Psychological patterns such as a sense of inferiority or helplessness that are associated with oppression clearly have their origin in social conditions of powerlessness and denigration … Such psychological patterns act as barriers to action and are part of what maintains oppression … Thus liberation must involve transformation of the psychological patterns as well as the social conditions associated with oppression" (Moane 2003: 92).

Methods and practice of liberation psychology.

Like popular education, liberation psychology seeks to ground itself in the "lived experience" of each group or community. As such, liberation psychology interventions will look different depending on the specific contexts of each group/community.

Moane (2003) and her colleagues utilize the person in environment/ecological model (Bronfenbrenner 1979; Trickett 1996) as a framework to identify the oppressive social conditions at the macro/cultural/institutional level that influence an individual's personal problems: (1) violence; (2) political exclusion; (3) economic exploitation; (4) control of sexuality; (5) cultural control; and (6) fragmentation. Any one of these patterns or experiences can adversely impact psychological well-being; in combination, they can create significant problems in the lives of those who are experiencing them (Moane 2003).

Liberation psychology practice involves addressing the psychological damage associated with oppression and empowering people to work to bring about change; Moane identifies change opportunities or liberation psychology practice opportunities at three levels: (1) facilitating personal development aimed at transforming patterns of internalized oppression and building strengths; (2) enabling individuals to work together in groups and communities; and (3) socio/political action: "accompanying" people and groups to take action to bring about change (Moane 2003).

Liberation psychology recognizes that many people may not be ready to engage with these opportunities until they have built up resources, skills and experience. A liberation psychology practitioner begins with the client's lived experience, and through dialogue and reflection, helps the client to develop a deeper and broader analysis and the confidence and skills necessary to do so (Belkin Martinez 2004; Freire 1974; Moane 2003).

Liberation psychology practice interventions might include supporting a client in developing the confidence to speak up at a meeting or helping a client obtain support from community groups or systems. At the political level, it might involve supporting a client's involvement in a particular movement for change (Belkin Martinez 2010; Moane 2003).

This understanding of the process of overcoming the psychological consequences of oppression is in keeping with Kieffer's (1984) developmental view of empowerment. He highlights the importance of allowing individuals and groups to "be in the driver's seat" around developing strategies for change. Other psychological frameworks which identify the connections between personal, interpersonal, and sociopolitical factors and psychological empowerment, or what Martín-Baró would call liberation, are the work of Morrow and Hawxhurst (1998) and Zimmerman's model of the components of personal empowerment (self-esteem, efficacy and capacity development) and collective behavior and action (Zimmerman 1990, 1995). Key to liberation psychology practice is the concept of solidarity with clients. Like Freire's learner/teacher, the liberation health practitioner is not the expert "treating" the client. Comas-Diaz, Lykes, and Alarcon (1998) talked about the concept of "accompanying" clients on their journey to liberation. Like Martín-Baró, they were critical of the role of a traditional psychologist and the stance of professional power and privilege/expertise. This concept of "accompanying" involves standing alongside people and working with them collaboratively.

The work of Rhea Almeida and her colleagues at the Institute of Family services in New Jersey is another example of a liberation psychology practice model. Almeida developed a "cultural context framework" which "presents clinical strategies that connect relational healing and liberation from the oppressive patterns that structure all institutions in our society, including communities, educational institutions, religious organizations workplaces, and families" (Almeida, Dolan-Del Vecchio, and Parker 2008: xiv). "Clients" or community members are engaged in a therapeutic process that involves self-reflection, worldview deconstruction, critical consciousness, solidarity, social education, and social action.

Radical social work/rank and file movement in the United States

"The profession of social work has never been able to rid itself of the ambiguity of hovering between an archaic individualism and a possibly radical collectivism" (Marvin Gettleman, in Reisch and Andrews 2002: 1). From its origins, the social work profession has mirrored the larger society's debates on the etiology of social and psychological problems and the most appropriate methods to address these problems (Ferguson 2009; Reisch and Andrews 2002). In their outstanding book summarizing the history of radical social work in the United States, Reisch and Andrews (202) outline the origins of the social work profession and the longstanding tension within the profession between an individually focused "case based" approach and a community/social action focus. Similar to its British counterparts, the dominant model of social work upon its inception was to provide relief or charity to the poor. Charity organization society social worker Mary Richmond, author of the book *Friendly Visiting Among the Poor* (1899), was instrumental in developing the "scientific case method" approach to "helping" the poor. Harkening back to the English Poor Laws and the concept of the "deserving poor," the scientific case method assessed the need for charity or aid, again distinguishing between the deserving and undeserving poor. As the profession further developed, the scientific case method was further refined to help social workers identify individual problems and design behavioral interventions (Ferguson 2009; Reisch and Andrews 2002; Richmond 1906).

In the context of this dominant model, a rich tradition of alternative social work community practice emerged, the most famous examples being the settlement house movement, of which Jane Adams' "Hull House" is the most well known. Settlement houses were not only concerned with helping immigrants integrate into American society and to adopt dominant US cultural values; their social workers also labored alongside immigrants to challenge inadequate working conditions and address other public health and safety issues. They did so recognizing the potential strength of low-income groups to identify mutual needs and achieve common goals (Reisch and Andrews 2002).

The writings and practice of Bertha Capen Reynolds helped to deepen and expand this community involvement tradition in US social work. At the start of her career, Reynolds worked as a psychiatric social worker with a focus on individual casework. However, through her ongoing practice with individuals, Reynolds came to believe that "society, not the client was pathological" (McQuaide 1987: 276). As Marxist theory began to inform her worldview, she started to question the relevance of social case work, wondering "will social work be the opiate of the people ... providing palliatives for a degree of misery that might become dangerous to the prevailing social order ... If the community is dominated by those who rule for exploitation, then social case work which serves the community would execute the designs of the ruling class and victimize clients" (Reynolds 1973: 126). She even questioned whether individual casework should be set aside until "a just social and healthy order is achieved" (Reynolds 1973: 123).

Instead of abandoning casework, Reynolds began to argue that organizing for social change should not be viewed as distinct from casework, but rather as an essential component of direct social work practice. She supported social work interventions that involved talking directly with clients about the socio-political factors affecting their lives and identified the concept of "active citizenship" as a method to engage individuals and families around more collective approaches to problems that beset individuals and communities. (Reynolds 1973; McQuaide 1987; Joseph 1986). Throughout the rest of her life, she continued to work toward a framework for practice that would include and combine Freudian and Marxist theories.

Reynolds, together with Mary Van Kleeck, was a prominent member of a vibrant movement of radical social workers that emerged in the United States in the 1930s and which has come to be known as the rank and file movement. This movement was actually a loose network of radical social workers across the nation with local groups in major urban centers including New York, Chicago, Philadelphia, Boston, St. Louis, Cleveland, Pittsburgh, Kansas City, Los Angeles, and San Francisco (Reisch and Andrews 2002).

Radical social workers supported economic planning, labor organizing and a wide range of social and political reforms. Some supported Franklin D. Roosevelt's (FDR) 1930s New Deal; others did not because they thought it was too limited. Rank and filers helped to develop the first social work unions and created their own journal, *Social Work Today*, which consistently published articles supporting progressive causes and promoting greater activism both inside and outside the social work profession (Reisch and Andrews 2002). The movement pressed social workers to adopt a "radical position and mission in American society" and was critical of individual casework which did not include a sociopolitical analysis (Selmi and Hunter 2001).

Some rank and file movement activists were avowed socialists and communists and pursued a more radical agenda, arguing that the capitalist social system of the United States needed to be replaced by a "democratic socialist society" (Hagen 1986: 726, in Reisch and Andrews 2002). In a speech to a National Conference of Social Work, for example, van Kleeck criticized FDR's New Deal for "preserving the profits of the corporate elite under the guise of improving the living standards of the common people" and cautioned that a "reliance upon government commits social work to the preservation of the status quo and separates them from their clients ... leading them into defense of the politicians in an effort to protect political institutions ... government is essentially dominated by the strongest economic power and becomes the instrument to serve the purposes of the groups possessing that power" (van Kleeck 1934: 475, in Reisch and Andrews 2002).

The influence of the rank and file movement declined significantly following World War II, and the marginalization and persecution of radical social workers during the Cold War years led to the movement's demise. Reynolds was forced to resign from Smith College's School of Social Work and was unable to secure another academic position (McQuaide 1987; Selmi and Hunter 2001; Reisch and

Andrews 2002). Radical social work did not reemerge until the late 1960s. Factors influencing this revival included the end of post-war economic growth, the growing global economic crisis and the emergence of new social movements beginning with the civil rights movement and spreading to the anti-war movement, the woman's movement, and the gay liberation movement (Ferguson 2009; Reisch and Andrews 2002).

Exposure to these radical social movements revived the earlier debates in the social work profession over the importance of social action and social justice struggles and their relationship to individually oriented models of casework, which were now increasingly seen as blaming individuals and families for their problems and minimizing the role of institutions and ideologies in contributing to personal problems (Reisch and Andrews 2002; Brake and Bailey 1980). In the United Kingdom, social work services were reconfigured based upon research studies about client experiences and new legislation in England and Scotland (Ferguson 2009). New books continued the critique of individualized casework and highlighted the role of oppression in creating and maintaining personal problems (Fergurson 2009; Brake and Bailey 1980; Corrigan and Leonard 1978; Bailey and Brake 1975).

As during the depression years, the radical social workers of the 1960s and 1970s were active both in new radical initiatives within the social work profession and as part of broader social movements. In the United Kingdom, radical social workers produced a magazine called *Case Con*, which challenged the traditional hierarchal relationships between workers and services users and called for alternative methods to conceptualize and intervene around identified problems, including political action and community work (Fergurson 2009). In the United States, radical social workers engaged in grassroots activism, community organizing, and radical study groups. Social workers were active in the National Welfare Rights Organization, La Raza, and Social Work Action for Human Rights (Reisch and Andrew 2002). Within the social work profession itself, the Social Welfare Worker's Movement (SWWM) was a social work organization which promoted a "socialist vision of a planned cooperative society" (Weinocur 1975: 3–4, quoted in Reisch and Andrews 2002). SWWM members placed a strong emphasis on community organizing and developed a five-point program for radical social work which focused on: "(1) decentralization and deprofessionalization; (2) exposure of social inequalities; (3) resistance to dehumanizing social welfare policies; (4) support for sweeping political and economic changes; and (5) coalition building with allies and alliances with client groups" (SWWM 1969, as quoted in Reisch and Andrews 2002).

The activities of radical social workers had a significant influence on the profession of social work. By the late 1960s, most national organizations supported the concept of social action as the "business of social work." The ideas of client self-determination, working collaboratively with families and communities, and conceptualizing problems as external to people became a large component of narrative and collaborative therapy models (Belkin Martinez 2004; Madsen 2007; Waldegrave, Tamasese, Thuaka, and Camphell 2003; White 2000). Yet as Reisch and

Andrew (2002) point out, the vast majority of social workers did not join radical organizations nor support radical tactics. Radical social work groups slowly disappeared and the tension between the rhetoric around social justice and actual clinical social work practice continued.

Methods and practice of radical social work

The radical social work tradition has left us a rich legacy of theoretical insights and practical methodology (Bailey and Brake 1975; Corrigan and Leonard 1978). Perhaps most important is its insistence that social activism is a legitimate form of social work practice. Reynolds, for example, did not view individual casework and community organizing as separate, distinct interventions since, for her, the problems of individuals and families were "beyond the scope of any one method" (Joseph 1986: 122).

In attempting to bridge the individual casework/social action tension, the Australian social worker Janis Fook (1993) produced an excellent text, *Radical Case Work*, which was specifically written for social workers who wanted to practice radical social work within a more traditional casework frame and setting. Drawing on socialist feminist theory for her conceptual framework, Fook identified five key elements of the radical social work casework: 1) A structural analysis of which personal problems can be traced to causes in the socio-political–economic structure; 2) an ongoing analysis of the social control functions of the social work profession and the social welfare system; 3) an ongoing critique of the existing social political and economic arrangements; 4) a commitment to protecting individuals against oppression by more powerful individuals, groups and structures; and 5) goals of personal liberation and social change (Fook 1993: 7).

Starting from this conceptual framework, Fook developed a system of assessment and intervention planning that included linking the personal problems of individuals with the structural problems of society, increasing awareness of how ideology influences a problem and enabling personal and social change (Fook 1993). Fook was clear that this process needs to be applied to both the theory and practice of casework and her book is one of the first texts that translates and applies broad concepts like ideology to specific techniques and intervention strategies. She does an excellent job extending traditional social work tasks, such as a focus on adjustment and coping, to an emphasis on helping an individual increase their control over the effects of institutions and social structures (Fook 1993). Fook's theory of practice, focused mostly on individual casework in Australia, is a seminal text for the radical social work clinician.

The liberation health model incorporates much of Fook's framework and expands the focus on developing a collaborative process of assessment and action planning with individuals, families, and communities. The liberation health framework also includes an activist component, which involves "rescuing the historic memory of change" (talking about examples in which ordinary people challenged external systems), and standing in solidarity with community members as they challenge ideological messages and institutions.

Liberation health theory and clinical practice

The liberation health social work model draws on, combines and further develops critical elements of the above three traditions to create a theory and approach to clinical practice for social work in the contemporary United States. Here are the broad elements of the liberation health model, which are further explained and illustrated in the other chapters in this volume.

General principles

Situating clients' problems in a social context

The liberation health model reaffirms the view that the problems of individuals, families and communities cannot be understood in isolation from the economic, political, cultural contexts in which they present themselves and from which they developed.

Social work has always had a "person in environment" orientation. Our code of ethics states: a "historic and defining feature of the social work is the profession's focus on individual well being in a social context and the well being of society. Fundamental to social work is attention to the environmental forces that create, contribute to, and address problems in living … social workers promote social justice and social change with and on behalf of individuals, families, groups, organizations, and communities" (National Association of Social Workers 2008).

While the vast majority of introductory social work textbooks begin with a summary of the NASW code of ethics preamble, as noted in our Introduction, there is a longstanding tension in the social work tradition on what this means in practice (Bailey and Brake 1975; Belkin Martinez 2004, 2005; Corrigan and Leonard 1978; Fook 1993; Reisch and Andrew 2002). The liberation health model explicitly reaffirms the importance for social workers to grasp the connections between the social conditions of an individual/family/community and their problems.

Reaffirming that social work practice must be both individual and social

The liberation health model is predicated upon the view that the solutions to the problems of individuals, families and communities must be both individual and social.

Liberation health argues that what are generally termed micro and macro practice do not need to be separate distinct interventions, but can and should be a parts of a singular integrated practice. Similar to Fook's casework model of radical social work and Almeida's cultural context framework, the liberation health model integrates individual case work with socio-political analysis and social action.

Recognizing the importance of ideology.

The liberation health model argues that ideology, how individuals, families and communities think about their problems and their relationships to them, is one of the most important arenas for critical social work practice.

In order to make sense of the world and their place in it, people need more than their direct perceptions; they need systems of meaning. Ideology, also called "worldview," provides groups and individuals with ideas, values and beliefs to guide their thinking and activities (Ferguson 2009; Saba 2004; Martín-Baró 1994; Fook 1993). "Everything, from how we think about God, life and death, to our choices about personal lifestyle and fashion reflect our worldview" (Saba 2004: 1). Ideology not only makes sense of the world, it also guides people in how they behave, what choices they make and how they judge their own behavior and that of others. The dominant ideological messages that we receive reflect the interests of the dominant class in a society (Saba 2004). For example, the ideological message of individualism – that individuals, not society, are responsible for their personal problems – reflects the interests of the dominant class. If institutions and social systems do not contribute to individuals' struggle with personal problems, then we do not need to reform or develop alternative institutions that might help these struggling individuals. By focusing on personal/familial roots of problems, we unwittingly collude in people's inclination to see their difficulties as reflections of their own inadequacies. In the same way, individualism and the lack of support for the idea of the government providing collective assistance to individuals is a significant impediment to the acceptance of a universal healthcare system for the United States.

How clients understand their problems and the ways they respond to them is rooted in their worldview. Liberation health social workers engage in ideological practice, that is, work with clients to expand the way they understand, analyze and respond to their problems as an essential precondition to effectively addressing them.

Changing consciousness, becoming subjects

Liberation health believes that effective social work practice involves working with clients to change their consciousness, to become "subjects" of their own life stories.

As noted earlier in the chapter, Paulo Freire wrote extensively about the effects of oppression on the human condition and described the effects of ongoing oppression as facilitating object-like experiences which impact an individual's self concept and sense of self efficacy" (Freire 1974). This passive sense of self is a serious obstacle that must be overcome if clients are going to make meaningful progress in addressing their problems. Liberation health insists that helping clients change their consciousness, transform their sense of self and become "subjects" capable of actively transforming their lives is key to effective social work practice.

The role of the social worker.

The liberation health model reaffirms the view that effective social work cannot be practiced as a top-down process of an "expert" providing solutions to grateful recipient clients, but must be a collaborative effort of allies. The North American psychologist William Madsen describes the preferred relational stance between client and therapist as that of an "appreciative ally stance in action" (Madsen 1999: 17). In his chapter on radical social work and service users, the British social work professor and service user Peter Beresford writes that the qualities of participatory, inclusive practice include: 1) the primacy of the relationship and human qualities in social work; 2) social work that is supportive and not controlling; 3) social work that involves co-production with service users; and 4) social work that ensures equal, diverse and inclusive involvement by all (Beresford 2011). For the liberation health social worker, this means our work with individuals, families and communities is a partnership which invites ways of thinking and acting that support and amplify client participation in the process; clients are in the "driver's seat" of all assessment and intervention/action planning.

Moreover, just as social workers collaborate alongside clients in understanding how ideology shapes the way they see their specific problems, so too, social workers must also struggle within the profession to see how ideology shapes the way the mental health system itself sees the world and where necessary, challenge and help to change it. Take the issue of "homosexuality," for example. Until 1987, ego dystonic homosexuality was identified as a diagnosis in the American Psychiatric Association's (APA) *Diagnostic and Statistical Manual of Mental Disorders* (DSM). The "knowledge" that homosexuality was an illness changed as a result of challenges to APA's classification system. Openly gay members of the APA and their allies staged a series of protests at annual conventions, culminating with an APA member testifying at a hearing with a clown mask on his face. The decision to remove ego dystonic homosexuality from the DSM occurred in the context of these massive protests (Bayer 1987). Beresford noted that effective social work is always political in nature: "If social work is functioning effectively with and on behalf of the individuals, families, groups and communities with whom it works, then it is likely to be challenging the market, both local and central state, and other powerful interests that may disempower them" (Beresford 2011: 106).

Methods and practice of liberation health social work

As noted earlier, both Freire and Martín-Baró were uneasy with prescribing general practice methods for their libratory initiatives. Liberation health practitioners share this unease. Nonetheless, there are some basic liberation health practice methods that can be broadly utilized when working with individuals, groups, families and communities if care is taken to tailor them to the specific populations involved. We will describe them in broad outline here. The following chapters provide specific examples of liberation health work in a variety of contexts and with a variety of populations.

Seeing a problem in its totality

Liberation health social work begins "where the client is at." In most cases, an individual or family problem or crisis initiates the referral for service. For the liberation health social worker, the first step is to develop a comprehensive view of the problem or crisis in collaboration with the client or clients. Martín-Baró and Freire called this seeing the problem in its totality (Freire 1996; Martín-Baró 1994). This process can have a number of steps involving a number of different techniques.

Seeing a problem in its totality is critical for liberation health practitioners because clients usually start out with a very limited or partial view of their problems, and this limited view is a critical impediment to developing the kinds of action plans necessary to address them. The job of the liberation health social worker is to partner with clients to progressively deepen, expand and transform their understanding of the nature, scope and dimensions of their problems and to question and rethink the terms in which they see them (and themselves) (Belkin Martinez 2005).

Working with clients to see problems in their totality starts with asking clients to describe the problem, the ways it has impacted their lives/family/ community, and how they (the clients) have dealt with it or similar problems in the past (Madsen 2007; White and Epston 1990). When working with groups or families, it is not uncommon for different family members to have different views of a problem or even to think that one or more members of the family are the problem itself (Madson 2007; White and Epston 1990). This initial identification of the problem or problems usually results in what the narrative therapist Michael White might call a "thin" description, a problem expressed in terms consistent with dominant worldview messages, values and prejudices. A liberation health social worker might start by asking each person to make a list of all the problems the family/group is experiencing. When everyone is finished, each individual shares their list of problems with the entire group; the group as a whole then discusses all of the identified problems and generates a list of common problems.

The next step is for the social worker to engage the client in a comprehensive analysis/rethinking of the problem. This is a collaborative effort to progressively deconstruct/transform the "thin" description of the problem and co-create a new "thicker" problem statement. A variety of techniques can be used in developing the new problem statement. One is to have the client create an external representation of the problem. This is sometimes called developing a code, or what Freire called a generative theme (Freire 1974) to represent the problem. Clients can create drawings, audio tapes, videos, a short theatre presentation or any other creative demonstration of the problem. This helps clients to externalize the problem and to look at it differently. Asking clients to draw their problem is a simple activity which helps facilitate a "thicker" description of the initial problem definition. Social workers can ask questions about the drawing which set the stage for a more complex multifactorial problem analysis. For example, an adolescent might initially describe the problem as "my mother … She is always on my back." As the adolescent draws this problem, the social worker asks additional problem posing questions: what exactly is going on when your mom is on your back, when does this happen, what do you say when this occurs, do you think there is something happening between you and your mom which leads to her being on your back? Seeing the problem in its totality through a drawing might facilitate a broader "thicker" definition of the initial problem. In the above example, the adolescent redefined the problem as "miscommunication."

For liberation health social workers, "problem analysis" is the next step in the development of the "thicker" problem statement. There are many methods of analyzing problems that are utilized in popular education and liberation psychology (Freire 1996). This casebook focuses on the use of a triangle, or triangulation of the problem. Triangulation involves placing the identified problem at the center of a triangle; the three points are identified as the personal, the cultural and the institutional factors influencing the problem. "Triangulating the problem" is a process of dialog between the social worker and the client or clients aimed at identifying, listing and describing all of the personal, cultural, and institutional factors that contribute or relate to the problem.

Martín-Baró referred to this process as "lifting the veil of ignorance" or problematization. Problematization is more than just adding additional information or factors to the "thin" description of the problem originally provided by the client. It is also a recursive method of questioning the narrative terms and taken-for-granted assumptions used in the client's initial description. It is a method of worldview deconstruction or "de-ideologizing" the client's original narrative (Belkin Martinez 2004, Martín-Baró 1994).

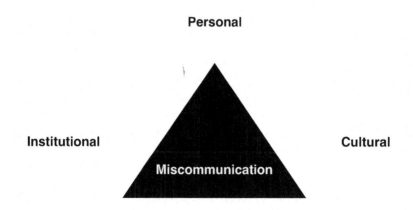

FIGURE 1.1 Liberation health theory and practice
Source: Dawn Belkin-Martinez

The liberation health social worker's role in this process is to help clients to think about the problem in new ways and in a much broader context. Ideally, in talking about their problem in a broader context of individual biological and social factors, cultural practices and messages, and institutions, clients begin to see their problems in a radically new light, to critically reflect on the language and assumptions they previously used to describe it, and to understand and narrate the problem in a new "thicker" and empowering way. On the basis of this new "thicker" description, a problem statement from which an action plan can be created is produced.

Developing and implementing an action plan

Based on the results of the collaborative effort to "see the problem in its totality" and analyze the personal, cultural and institutional factors contributing to the problem, liberation health social workers and clients then collaborate to develop comprehensive action plans to address the problem. These action plans become the basic working tools which then guide the relationship between social worker and client for the remainder of their collaboration.

For many clients, the action plan can take the form of a simple four column chart which is updated weekly: column #1: the various aspects of the problem; column #2: what needs to change in relation to each; column #3: the long range vision or goal in relation to each; and column #4: specific activities and initiatives for week (Belkin Martinez 2004).

Because the problem was ultimately identified and described in all its dimensions, personal, cultural and institutional, the action plan likewise usually includes specific actions and activities in all these dimensions. This can mean taking action around a personal factor, such as helping someone cope with their anxiety by creating an affect management plan, challenging cultural messages by deconstructing dominant ideas about gender or race, or taking action on an institutional front such as attending a take back the night march or going to a community protest against gentrification. While action plans are often initially focused on the personal factors affecting a problem, the liberation health social worker introduces questions and observations related to the cultural and institutional factors contributing to the problem. For example, while a young Latino male might be working on behavioral techniques to decrease his aggressive behavior, a liberation health social worker might introduce questions about the role racism plays in the identified problem. The client and worker might read up on current events together and explore opportunities to be involved in anti-racist activities in the community.

The action plan and its various components are reviewed and, if necessary, revised, and updated weekly. This process, which Freire referred to as praxis, is a recursive and iterative process involving action, reflection, action. Through action plans and clients' reflections on them and what they are able to achieve as the plan progresses, liberation health social work helps them to recover subject-like experiences and memories of when clients, and members of their community were able to affirmatively act in the world. This is what is sometimes referred to as "rescuing the historical memory of change" (Almeida, Dolan-Del Vecchio, and Parker 2008; Belkin Martinez 2005; Fook 1993; Freire 1974; Martín-Baró 1994). The ultimate goal is to facilitate the transition of clients from objects to subjects and to not only enable them to master and overcome the problem or crisis which brought them into the social work system, but to be better able to deal with future problems or crises which might arise in their lives.

Liberation health social work resources

There are a number of resources nationally and internationally that make use of the liberation health model and similar theories and practice methods. These include the following:

- **Boston Liberation Health Group**: The Boston Liberation Health Group (BLHG) is committed to addressing the structural and institutional flaws in our healthcare system and its refusal to recognize healthcare as a fundamental human right. BLHG acts: 1) as a support group for healthcare professionals working to bring social justice issues into their direct practice with clients; 2) as a peer supervision group for individuals and groups practicing the methods of liberation health in their work; and 3) politically in the communities in which we live and work, standing in solidarity with other organizations and individuals working for social justice (source: liberationhealth.org).
- **The Radical Social Work Group**: The Radical Social Work Group (RSWG) is a group of activist social workers based in New York City who are committed to social change and to developing a praxis for radical social work. The RSWG seeks to: 1) dismantle oppressive institutions and injustice; 2) do work that goes to the root of problems and "changes them from there"; and 3) do what they can within the system to change how the system has historically worked. Retrieved May 6th 2013 from http//sites.google.com/site/radicalswg
- **Rank and Filer**: The Rank and Filer is a weekly blog for people working in social services that provides political analysis for radical social workers. This blog shares histories of radical social movements and events and posts articles for people working in medical care, non profits, welfare departments and community organizing projects (source: rankandfiler.net).
- **Bay Area Mutual Aid**: Bay Area Mutual Aid is a group of social workers committed to fighting for social justice in our communities, workplaces and society at large, by organizing and mobilizing social workers, supporting each other, and collaborating with other professionals, clients, and community stakeholders. We apply a broad definition to the title "social worker" and seek to engage all those doing social work in its many forms. We believe that social change and social justice are integral to all forms of social work and hope to reinvigorate out field's commitment to and understanding of "social change and social justice." Instead of looking away from abuses of power, we seek to apply

a critical understanding of power, privilege and oppression to our work (source: bayareamutualaid.org).

- **Social Work Action Network**: The Social Work Action Network (SWAN) is a radical campaigning organization of social work practioners, students, service users, carers and academics. SWAN is based in the UK, but has international chapters. Its main objective is to promote a social work practice which is rooted in the value of social justice, which seeks to advocate alongside and on behalf of carers and service users and which values both individual relationship based practice and collective approaches. SWAN strives to strengthen the radical voice within social work practice, education, and wider policy debates (source: socialworkfuture.org).

- **Social Welfare Action Alliance**: The Social Welfare Action Alliance (SWAA) is a national organization of progressive social workers based in the United States. SWAA seeks to: 1) promote the study and practice of the progressive tradition in social welfare policy by critiquing the nature of social services, social work and social change; 2) understand the methods of humanistic direct practice that supports individual, community, and broad social change; and 3) promote the participation of social service workers in the struggles of low income and other oppressed people (source: socialwelfareactionalliance.org).

- **Institute for Family Services**: The Institute for Family Studies applies Rhea Almeida's cultural context model approach to social work practice. The cultural context model is a sociopolitical model of family therapy which links social justice to all levels of family therapy. Key concepts include accountability, critical consciousness, cultural circles, empowerment, and understanding the connections between the multiple layers of oppression (intersectionality) (Almeida, Dolan-Del Vecchio, and Parker2008).

Critical and Radical Social Work Journal: *Critical and Radical Social Work* is an international journal that seeks to analyze and respond to issues such as the impact of global neoliberalism on social welfare, austerity and social work, and social movements and inequality and oppression (source: www.policypress.co.uk/journals_crsw_aas.asp?).

References

Aambo, A. (1997) Tasteful solutions: Solution-focused work with groups of immigrants. *Contemporary Family Therapy*, 19 (1): 63–79.

Almeida, R. V., Dolan-Del Vecchio, K., and Parker, L. (2008) *Transformative Family Therapy: Just Families in a Just Society*. Boston, MA: Pearson Education.

Bailey, R. and Brake, M. (eds) (1975) *Radical Social Work*. New York: Pantheon.

Bartlett, L. (2005) Dialogue, knowledge and teacher-student relations: Freirean pedagogy in theory and practice. *Comparative Education Review*, 49 (5): 344–64.

Bayer, R. (1987) *Homosexuality and American Psychiatry: The Politics of Diagnosis*. Princeton, NJ: Princeton University Press.

Belkin Martinez, D. (2004) Therapy for liberation: The Paulo Freire methodology. Available online at http://liberationhealth.org/documents/freiresummarysimmons.pdf (accessed October 1, 2013).

Belkin Martinez, D. (2005) Mental healthcare after capitalism. *Radical Psychology*, 4 (2). Available online at www.radicalpsychology.org/vol4-2/Martinez4.html (accessed October 1, 2013).

Belkin Martinez, D. (2010) Solidaridad y justicia: Latinas, community organizing, and empowerment. In R. Furman and N. Negi (eds), *Social Work Practice with Latinos: Key Issues and Emerging Themes*, chapter 17. Chicago, IL: Lyceum Books.

Beresford, P. (2011) Radical social work and service users: A crucial connection. In M. Lavalette (ed.), *Radical Social Work Today: Social Work at the Crossroads*. Bristol: Policy Press, pp. 95–114.

Brake, M. and Bailey, R. (eds) (1980) *Radical Social Work and Practice*. London: Edward Arnold.

Breton, M. (1994) On the meaning of empowerment and empowerment – Oriented social work practice. *Social Work with Groups*, 17 (13): 23–37.

Bronfenbrenner, U. (1979) *The Ecology of Human Development*. Cambridge, MA: Harvard University Press.

Burton, M. and Kagan, C. (2005) Liberation social psychology: Learning from Latin America. *Journal of Community and Applied Psychology*, 15: 63–78.

Castano, E., Castano, F., and Paulo, J. (1993) A practical application of popular education techniques [Workshop handout]. Brecht Forum, New York.

Comas-Diaz, L, Lykes, M. B., and Alarcon, R. D. (1998) Ethnic conflict and the psychology of liberation in Guatemala, Peru, and Puerto Rico. *American Psychologist*, 53 (7): 778–91.

Corrigan, P. and Leonard, P. (1978) *Social Work Practice Under Capitalism: A Marxist Approach*. London: Macmillian.

Fanon, F. (1967) *The Wretched of the Earth*. London: Penguin.

Ferguson, I. (2009) Another social work is possible: Reclaiming the radical tradition. In V. Leskosek (ed.), *Theories and Methods of Social Work: Exploring Different Perspectives*. Ljubljana, Slovenia: Faculty of Social Work, University of Ljubljana, pp. 81–98.

Freire, P. (1970, 2003) *Pedagogy of the Oppressed*. New York: Continuum International.

Freire, P. (1974) Education as the practice of freedom. In: Education for critical consciousness, London, UK: Continuum [Original work published 1968], pp. 1–78.

Fook, J. (1993) *Radical Casework: A Theory of Practice*. St. Leonards, NSW: Allen and Unwin.

Freire, P. (1998) *Pedagogy of Freedom: Ethics, Democracy, and Civic Courage*. Latham, MD: Rowman and Littlefield.

Freire, P. (1996) *Letters to Christina: Reflections of My Life And Work*. London: Routledge.

Hagen, J. (1986) Mary van Kleeck. In W. Trattner (ed.), *Biographical Dictionary of Social Welfare in America*. Westport, CT: Greenwood, pp. 725–8.

Hegar, R. (2012) Paulo Freire: Neglected mentor for social work. *Journal of Progressive Human Services*, 23 (2): 159–77.

hooks, b. (1993) *Sisters of the Yam: Black women and Self-recovery*. Boston, MA: South End Press.

Joseph, B. (1986) The Bertha C. Reynolds centennial conference June 28–30, 1985: Taking organizing back to the people. *Smith College Studies in Social Work*, 56 (2): 122–31.

Kieffer, C. (1984) Citizen empowerment: A developmental perspective. In J. Rapport and R. Hess (eds), *Studies in Empowerment: Steps Toward Understanding and Action*. New York: Haworth Press, pp. 9–36.

Kline, M., Dolgon, C., and Dresser, L. (2000) The politics of knowledge in theory and practice: Collective research and political action in grassroots community organization. *Journal of Community Practice*, 8 (2): 23–32.

Madsen, W. (1999, 2007) *Collaborative Therapy with Multi-Stressed Families: From Old Problems to New Futures*. New York: Guilford Press.

Martín-Baró, I. (1994) *Writings for a Liberation Psychology: Essays 1985–1989*. A. Aron, and S. Corne (eds). Cambridge, MA: Harvard University Press.

McQuaide, S. (1987) Beyond the logic of pessimism: A personal portrait of Bertha Capen Reynolds. *Clinical Social Work Journal*, 3, 271–80.

Moane, G. (2003) Bridging the personal and the political: practices for a liberation psychology. *American Journal of Community Psychology*, 31 (1/2): 91–101.

Moane, G. (2010) Sociopolitical development and political activism: Synergies between feminist and liberation psychology. *Psychology of Women Quarterly*, 34: 521–9.

Montero, M. and Sonn, C. (eds) (2009) *The Psychology of Liberation: Theory and Applications*. New York: Springer.

Morrow, S. L. and Hawxhurst, D. M. (1998) Feminist therapy: Integrating political analysis in counseling and psychotherapy. *Women and Therapy*, 21 (2): 37–50.

National Association of Social Workers (2008) Code of ethics of the National Association of Social Workers. Available online at www.socialworkers.org/pubs/code/code.asp (accessed October 1, 2013).

Reisch, M. and Andrews, J. (2002) *The Road Not Taken: A History of Radical Social Work in the United States*. London: Brunner-Routledge.

Reynolds, B. (1973) *Between Client and Community*. New York: Oriole Press.

Richmond, M. E. (1899) *Friendly Visiting Among the Poor: A Handbook for Charity Workers*. New York: Macmillan.

Richmond, M. E. (1906) *Industrial Conditions and the Charity Worker*. Mary Richmond Collection. New York: Columbia University.

Saba, P. (2004) Worldview for activists: An introduction. Boston, MA: Liberation Health Group. Available online at www.liberationhealth.org/documents/Worldview forOrganizers5_2__2_.pdf (accessed October 1, 2013).

Selmi. P. and Hunter, R. (2001) Beyond the rank and file movement: Mary van Kleeck and social work radicalism in the Great Depression, 1931–1942. *Journal of Sociology and Social Welfare*, 25: 75–100.

Torres, C. A. and Fischman, G. (1994) Popular education: Building from experience. *New Directions for Adult and Continuing Education*, 63: 81–93.

Trickett, E. J. (1996) A future for community psychology: The contexts of diversity and the diversity of contexts. *American Journal of Community Psychology*, 24: 209–35.

van Kleeck, M. (1934) Our Illusions Regarding Government (Pugsley Award). *Proceedings of the National Conference on Social Work*, 61st Annual Session. Chicago: University of Chicago Press, pp. 428–37.

Waldegrave, C., Tamasese, K., Tuhaka, F., and Campbell, W. (2003) *Just Therapy: A Journey. A Collection of Papers from the Just Therapy Team, New Zealand*. Adelaide: Dulwich Centre Publications.

White, M. (2000) *Reflections on Narrative Practice*. Adelaide: Dulwich Centre Publications.

White, M. and Epston, D. (1990) *Narrative Means to Therapeutic Ends*. New York: Norton.

Zimmerman, M. A. (1995) Psychological empowerment: Issues and Illustrations. *American Journal of Community Psychology*, 23 (5): 581–99.

Zimmerman, M. A. (1990) Toward a theory of learned hopefulness: A structural model analysis of participation and empowerment. *Journal of Research in Psychology*, 24: 71–86.

2

BECOMING A LIBERATION HEALTH SOCIAL WORKER

Jared Douglas Kant

Introduction

This chapter presents the writer's experience of a transformative process that began at the beginning of graduate school and carried through into post-school clinical practice. It is largely written in the first person, and seeks to outline a process of self-awareness and self-actualization that is essential to the training of liberation health-based social workers. The case study will cover a social worker's entrance into formal training, the confrontation of class privilege and the introduction of new information that challenged this writer's worldview. *Formulation* and *intervention* are used in a non-traditional way in this context, referring to different stages of a single process of transformation. While this process will look different in all students, there are aspects that can be applied universally. Liberation health requires that practitioners not be casual, passive observers of systems of oppression. It asks and demands that clinicians engage in a dialog with these systems and the communities that they burden. The intervention section offers, as an example one worker's confrontation of his own socialization, privilege and education.

Literature review

The chapter begins with an overview of some of the central literature that has informed the writer's understanding of his experience. While all of this is viewed from the perspective of liberation health, many different fields have contributed to the de-pathologization of mental health care and the refocus on environmental (cultural and institutional) factors that maintain what is seen by conventional discourse as "pathology" (Almeida, Dolan-Del Vecchio, and Parker 2007). Some of these contributions come from disparate fields covering seemingly unrelated topics, including but not limited to: labor struggle, educational theories, immigration, and neurobiology. Throughout the body of the text, readers will find references to literature whose explicit incorporation into the text is beyond the scope of the chapter.

Liberation health mandates that practitioners heed the historical moment of our clients. This requires being sensitive to greater social and political discourses that intersect with our clients' own, unique lives (Martín-Baró, Aron, and Corne 1994). To understand and engage in liberatory therapy therefore requires a reconstruction of the understanding of the relationship of the therapist to practice (ibid, p. 38). Martín-Baró adopted this idea from the work of Paulo Friere, who stated that for liberatory teaching, the "teacher-student contradiction be resolved," where teachers are also students and students are also teachers (Friere 2000: 66). Freire emphasized the resolution of this dichotomy because he envisioned that teachers should learn from their own students' experiences, and elicit the curriculum from them, rather than assume expert status (ibid, p. 67).

To fully engage in liberatory practice, practitioners must first grapple with the dominant stories in their own lives that may be affecting their practice (Almeida, Dolan Del-Vecchio, Parker 2007). The task is two-fold: first, confronting one's own privilege as a professional; and second, joining in the process of struggle with the communities in question. Examples of this can be found across disciplines from education, to medicine, to history and psychology.

In a conversation with David Barsamian, Howard Zinn said that he felt the most important teaching he did was outside of the classroom, standing in solidarity with protesting students during his short tenure at Spelman College (Zinn and Barsamian 1999). In other works, Zinn describes having come to this place of action after confronting the selective nature of material in his own profession, where industrialists were glamorized, and pioneer feminists and anarchist thinkers, like Emma Goldman, were completely ignored. Zinn wanted to teach a view of history that celebrated acts of resistance, to offer hope.

In writing about liberatory education, Freire wrote that liberatory education could only be achieved through praxis: the simultaneous discussing and doing, where the discussion shapes the action and vice-versa (Freire 2003). Liberatory therapy asks the worker to engage the social issues of contention directly, rather than from afar. For this, liberation health calls for workers to become clinician activists.

Clinician activists are not new to the field of mental health. Harvard psychiatrist Matthew Dumont famously organized speak-outs in front of the press, and facilitated the forming of community coalitions made up of members that were most affected by oppressive policies (Dumont 1994). He describes coming to this after a realization that his work as a community psychiatrist was "at odds" with the dominant discourse of mainstream psychiatry (ibid, p. 9). It is thus that Dumont engages in this same process, first challenging professional discourse and then challenging the oppressive systems themselves, this time aligned with his community of service in Chelsea, Massachusetts.

Social work pioneer Bertha Capen Reynolds writes in her autobiography about the radicalization many social workers experienced trying to reconcile practicing psychiatric casework without tending to the complete lack of resources impacting their clients (Reynolds 1991: 138). It was at this time that Reynolds writes hearing reports from other social workers of eviction blockades and actions to prevent foreclosure auctions (ibid, p. 154). Reynolds herself became an active member of the labor movement, seeing the need for economic justice as inextricably linked to the aims of social work. Seeking explanations for social ills that existed outside of the internal world of clients, Reynolds brought Marxism to social work education and became involved in what is now known as the "rank and file movement," a coalition of social workers who sought to bridge political consciousness with clinical practice (ibid, p. 158).

David Gil, a professor of social work at Brandeis University recounts his own struggles with recognizing the "contradictions, limitations and futility of clinically oriented social services" (Reisch and Andrews 2001). To take his clinical ideals to their logical conclusion, Gil ultimately became the co-chair of the Socialist Party USA (ibid, p. 219) to advocate for greater systemic change.

Social workers, perhaps more than any other professional, are called upon to respond to situations steeped in systems of oppression (McGoldrick 1998). The social worker at the prison must confront disproportionality in sentencing and the pipeline-to-prison that has claimed so many youth (Christensen 2012). The community health worker in predominately immigrant communities must acknowledge and confront the truth that *hypervigilance* can be explained as much by authoritarian Immigration and Customs Enforcement (ICE) raids in the middle of the night as it can by trauma survived in countries of origin (Capps, Castañeda, Chaudry, and Santos 2007; McLeigh 2010). With no exceptions, clinical situations are back to back with greater socio-political issues (Dumont 1992, 1994). In these instances, workers must consider taking practice outside of the session to the socio-political realm of activism (ibid).

To enter into a clinician activist role requires the first step of confronting one's own relative place in the web of privilege. The process of confronting one's own privilege is explored by Harro (2000), who writes that "We need to take a stand, reframe our understandings, question the status quo, and begin a critical transformation that can break down this cycle of socialization and start a new cycle leading to liberation for all" (Harro 2000, p. 21).

Harro writes that systems of privilege create the roles of *agents and targets*. Agent roles are those that facilitate privilege, such as being white or male. While no one actively has a choice into which role they are born, by not engaging into reflection on their agent status, people become complicit in the oppression of those in subordinate, or *target* roles (ibid, p. 19).

Many bodies of thought were critical to the transformation of the author and the author's understanding of the communities in which he found himself. These will be presented in citation throughout the text.

The remainder of this chapter will be written in the first person.

Case study

As a first year social work intern, it became apparent to me that my social work education would take me outside of the confines of academia and even beyond the confines of the clinic. To truly engage in liberatory practice, I concluded that I first had to challenge my own worldview and immerse myself in experiences that were radically different from that with which I was already familiar.

Drawn by the romanticization of the criminal justice system in popular discourse, I had asked that my first placement in graduate school be in a forensic setting. I interviewed and had been placed at a juvenile court clinic in Suffolk County, located inside a large courthouse in the center of Boston.

My principle function as a court clinician intern was to assess juveniles, who had been referred either by a judge or probation officer, for potential mental health issues that might underlie the behaviors for which they were before the court. By and large, my clients had been charged with "status offenses," which means that what they had done was prohibited by their status as minors. The classifications included truancy, running away, school disruptions and even stubbornness, in what is known as a "CHINS Stubborn Child" petition. Unlike a criminal offense, these were not actions that could land a juvenile in jail, but could lead to removal from their families of origin or being placed in psychiatric or state care.

There are literally endless reasons why a child or teenager might find themselves in front of a court clinician. Within the first two weeks of reviewing case files and observing court proceedings, I began to develop a tremendous unease about the fundamental unfairness of the situations in which clients found themselves.

Having worked previously in manual-driven psychiatric research, I had never before worked with clients who were facing the situations that had contributed to these young people's coming before the court. Families trying to make every dollar count, living below the radar of immigration enforcement, were struggling to fit two 40-hour jobs per parent into a schedule. Children were growing up in communities saturated with gangs and foreclosures, with little guarantee moment to moment of personal safety.

My supervisor at the time was a veteran of the Department of Mental Health, and had been conducting clinical and forensic interviews with clients for decades. Exasperated and feeling confused, I relayed to her an exchange between myself and a client. We had been going back and forth about his community, and I was constructing a map of his neighborhood in my head. From what I understood, my client lived with his mother on the first floor of a duplex, in a predominately Spanish-speaking neighborhood in the northern part of the greater Boston area. The neighborhood he lived in was part residential and part industrial. Much of Boston's manufacturing and shipping industries are concentrated in a relatively small portion of the city, making for peculiar geography and pronounced racial and class divisions. A boy of about ten, my client turned to me after thinking over one of my questions and stated, with no trace of irony or disingenuity: "We thought there was a gun, so we did what we always do. You know how it is. You get on the floor on your stomach like the army crawl, so the bullets don't hit you if they come through the glass."

After I recounted this, my supervisor smiled at me, and said simply "Yes, this isn't a suburban community. You need to learn that." While we often did not see eye-to-eye, she was not wrong. I had no context for this sort of experience. As the need for such a context grew, so did a deconstruction of the dominant messages I had been subject to, regarding living in socioeconomic distress. Furthermore, it was increasingly apparent that my own upbringing was wrought with privilege, and provided an inadequate context for understanding the lives of my clients.

Later in the chapter, I will address how to challenge *dominant discourse*, also known as *dominant worldview*. Liberation-centered practitioners have long empha-sized the need for therapists to heed their own privilege, understood from many different dimensions of race, religion, geospatial/geographic location, sexual orientation, biological/assigned gender, gender identity and class (Almeida, Dolan Del-Vecchio, Parker 2007: 32).

Towards the end of the year, I was working at my desk and received word from a colleague at a public school in Chelsea that a client had been arrested by school police for "trespassing" in a different school. When I asked where the other school was located, my colleague explained that it was actually the same building as the school he was supposed to be in, but that he had chosen to go for a walk and had strayed into the other school's classrooms. For the next couple of hours, I conducted an interview on the concrete floor in the basement of a courthouse, where holding cells were set up for detainees awaiting a hearing, talking to a client in his pre-teenage years who was behind plated bulletproof glass and bars.

As we alternated between talking and silence, constantly alert to the relative lack of privacy afforded by his cell, I came full face to the reality that never in my near two decades of youthful indiscretion, had I risked being in the situation of my interviewee. Children in the areas I was serving and, indeed, in many underprivileged communities across the United States, are facing an onslaught of zero-tolerance legislation, side by side with other social realities (Kupchik 2010). This boy was the son of a mother who had escaped domestic violence by immigrating to the United States. He had to bear his mother's fears about living in this country with the tenuous "undocumented status" and what that entailed when interacting with figures in authority. Without adequate work opportunities, his mother was struggling to get by on her overwhelming work schedule and could not afford private representation for my client, nor was she able to advocate for the state to provide such a service itself. Only racism, xenophobia, and the disparate wealth distribution of US capitalism could explain the difference between my prior situation and his. It was a lesson that contributed to a feeling that any interventions I may hope to use as a traditional therapist would be irrelevant in a larger context of oppression and inequality unless I found a way to bring conversations about oppression into the clinical session.

It was at this time that I identified most specifically a feeling of general unease that appeared whenever I found myself attempting to put practice knowledge into actual practice.

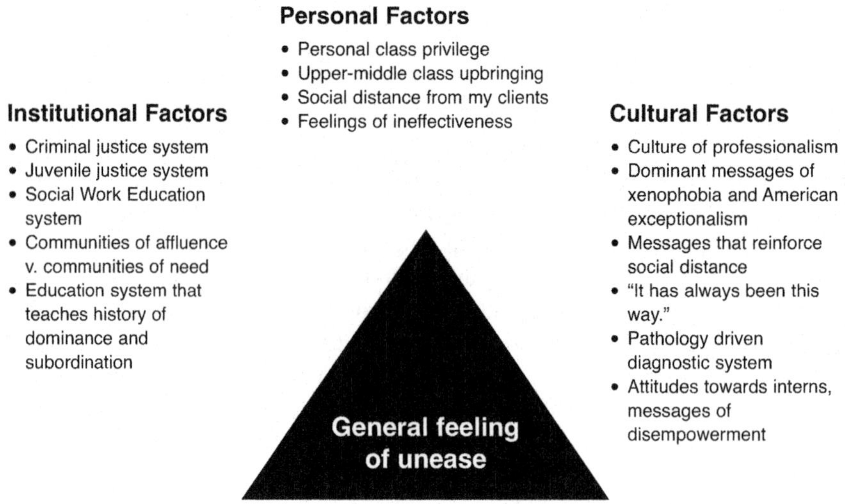

Personal Factors

- Personal class privilege
- Upper-middle class upbringing
- Social distance from my clients
- Feelings of ineffectiveness

Institutional Factors

- Criminal justice system
- Juvenile justice system
- Social Work Education system
- Communities of affluence v. communities of need
- Education system that teaches history of dominance and subordination

Cultural Factors

- Culture of professionalism
- Dominant messages of xenophobia and American exceptionalism
- Messages that reinforce social distance
- "It has always been this way."
- Pathology driven diagnostic system
- Attitudes towards interns, messages of disempowerment

General feeling of unease

FIGURE 2.1 Becoming a liberation health social worker
Source: Jared Kant

Much as family therapists may say that working with a client without bringing the family into the room is incomplete (Minuchin, Colapinto, and Minuchin 2007), working with a family without bringing the greater institutions and cultural factors into the room is also incomplete (Almeida, Dolan-Del Vecchio, and Parker 2007). Therefore, one goal of liberation health practice is to bring conversations around macro systems into the room. However, the limits to what can be achieved inside the walls of therapy demands that social workers be agents of change outside the office. Therefore, clinical practice is complimented by bringing the knowledge clients hold to help inform struggles in the community and society. These two processes of macro and micro work inform each other.

Given what I had come to understand about the population I was working with, and as the National Association of Social Workers code of ethics explicitly states that the social worker must be most sensitive to the most marginalized of clients, it had become explicitly clear to me that my work needed to go beyond the confines of individual or family sessions or the most scrupulous of reports. I have found this principle consistently reaffirmed in every subsequent practice environment since that first year as an intern.

The following year, I found myself at a new internship, a school. The school where I was placed was a residential treatment facility for children. As in the court, these children struggled with enormous challenges made that much greater by the cycle of systemic oppression.

While classroom learning would suggest that children who had experienced multiple disrupted foster placements required consistency and predictability, budget constraints precluded the ability of providers to make this clinical wisdom into reality. Children who were academically successful for the first time in several years faced returning to the same system that had been unsuccessful in meeting their learning needs only a year before. This was a natural consequence of state and local government austerity measures, whereby funds were cut from social services to underwrite the financial irresponsibility and social disregard of the major corporate interests that shape public policy around the distribution of tax dollars.

What I felt I had begun to witness could have been described easily as colonialism. Colonialism is a system where one group in a position of power imposes its will on a subject group, robbing that group of necessary resources, devastating the community. Take this historical moment in the city of Boston as context for my entry into the role of social worker (taken from my personal journal, in italics for emphasis):

> *While the residents of more affluent communities were not invading the streets of Roxbury with armadas, the affluent way of life was being maintained by reckless budget cuts and foreclosures. As foreclosures in Dorchester increased, so did parental stress. As parental stress increased, so did "family dysfunction." Simultaneously, as cuts pervaded the Massachusetts budget, so did premature discharges from mental health facilities and inappropriate school placements. Residential placements can cost upwards of ten times the amount required for an in-district placement. As districts failed to produce testing results commensurate with Department of Education standards, public schools were being auctioned off to private companies who founded Charter schools in their place.*
>
> *Parents who wanted their children to attend the better-funded charter schools had to enter their children in a lottery system. Social work jobs in the Boston Public Schools were subcontracted out to private organizations. As a result of this increase in privatization, school-testing scores obtained a new status as viable predictors of success, as greater scores determined greater access. This strengthened the divide of classism, a cultural factor that greatly underscores institutional factors, such as class and race-based sentencing disparities in criminal cases.*

Both the children in the court clinic and the students at the residential school were identified as having psychiatric issues that contributed to the problems for which they were seeking assessment and treatment. Personal factors such as "attention-deficit hyperactivity disorder" and "major depressive disorder" were seen as existing alone in a systemic vacuum. As a liberation health practitioner, my job was to recognize that children who present as clinically depressed may also be struggling with the impact of external systems on their world (Almeida, Dolan Del-Vecchio, Parker 2007: 22). For example, they might be missing loved ones who were lost to community violence, worrying about parents overstretched by multiple jobs or lacking access to sufficient housing and food resources. The omnipresence of law enforcement may offer additional stress. Children may register increased police presence to signify greater danger, and stress response systems (the parts of our brain responsible for letting us know that we are in danger) may be constantly triggered, resulting in the symptom clinicians call hypervigilance: police presence may signify greater danger and threat, rather than safety or reassurance. As colonialism continues to drain communities of their essential resources, stress increases and bolsters pre-existing personal, cultural and institutional factors that contribute to what we call "mental illness."

What I was learning was that cultural messages and institutions were colluding to systematically disempower my clients and the communities from which they came. The name for a system where multiple forces of oppression act in such a way as to preserve power for the powerful and to continue to deny power to the disempowered is hegemony. In essence, I began to suspect that in addition to the liberation that occurred within my clinical practice, I had an ethical mandate to combat hegemony without.

It is in this vortex of intersecting systems of oppression that new students and practitioners of social work find themselves thrown, almost from the start. Despite these sometimes glaring overlaps between personal, cultural and institutional factors, dominant messages of individual deficit and dysfunction still pervade mental health education. My primary tools of assessment and diagnosis focused on internal struggles, but did not offer solutions for rectifying the greater social and cultural ills that played key parts in producing the very distress for which a client might present in a clinic. For this, it was clear that my clinical practice had to extend outside the clinic and outside of individual work. To be able to work towards a socially just society, I had to engage myself in political struggle. As well, it was critical that I engage myself in the practice of asking myself key questions about that which I had accepted thus far as truth with respect to diagnosing and understanding problems associated with mental health.

Intervention

The presenting problem, as thus outlined, is two-fold. First, I felt that the tools (specifically the language) I had been given in social work school were inadequate to properly describe the experiences of my clients. I found myself struggling with unhelpful discourses that pathologized clients and blamed the victims of oppression for their own struggles. Second, I had come to realize that the process of liberatory practice required that I immerse myself in the struggles that affected my clients.

To address these two major concerns, I set three important goals:

1. Address the "feeling of unease" through deconstruction of dominant discourse. Where was this feeling of unease coming from? What was making me uneasy? Could this unease within myself be traced to larger systemic issues?
2. Learn about and engage in the active struggle against all axes of oppression with particular attention to immigration, race, and economic justice.
3. Challenge the notion that oppressive systems are permanent and unchangeable: that this is "just how things are."

Deconstructing dominant discourse

The process of becoming aware of the dominant discourse that shaped my professional understanding of mental health was a dramatic first step in my transformation as a clinician activist. As the first step to liberation, it represented a process that Martín-Baró would name "*De-ideologizing everyday experience*" (Martín-Baró, Aron and Corne 1994: 31). The fundamental idea is that everyday experience is not neutral, but is shaped by "ideology." That means, the way we understand our daily life experiences is influenced and shaped by messages that we have been given as part of our socialization.

"De-ideologizing" or challenging "dominant discourse" involves breaking down these messages into their essential components and challenging the veracity of each sub-component. Identifying dominant discourse allows you to identify world views that support hegemony (see above for definition). These stories often marginalize an already oppressed group, or provide justification for the existence of stereotypes, social stigmas and other cultural messages of oppression. For example, the meaning that we may make as social workers of a cluster of symptoms is likely constructed by our understanding of theAmerican Psychological Association *Diagnostic and Statistical Manual of Mental Disorders* (DSM). The DSM teaches that problems are clusters of symptoms that present themselves in clients, and that these problems exist within clients. Learning to separate an individual's experience from his or her diagnosis allows us to see the problem in its totality.

As discussed at length in the previous section, I had discovered that my experiences as a white, upper-middle-class male put me in a particular social vantage point that made it difficult for me to access the realities of my clients. As I can no more shirk my whiteness or privilege than I can the experiences that drove me to social work school in the first place, it was important to find an alternative method of deconstructing, challenging and expanding my world view. To do so, one first must identify *dominant discourse*.

Challenging dominant discourse involves asking key questions about information being presented. Some of these questions include:

- Would I experience this information differently if I possessed a different social vantage point?
- In whose interest is it that I know this information?
- Who is telling me this information, and why are they telling the story the way that they are telling it?

In my experience at the court, I had discovered that my understanding of the politics of immigrant rights was inadequate. When I asked myself the questions as listed above, in relation to the question "What do I know about immigrant rights?," I discovered several shocking characteristics. All stories I found were told from a single vantage point. Each story was written from the perspective of an insider citizen, watching and musing about the struggles of outsiders attempting to gain access to the United States. Each story was written with the assumption that crossing the border was an act of moral transgression, resulting in inevitable job losses and tax burdens.

After identifying the manner in which immigration news stories in the United States were typically told, I sought media outlets that told the story from alternative viewpoints. Alternative media here will be defined as media that is produced by a non-dominant group and not for the sake of profit. These outlets will prefer multiple vantage points, and hope to elicit information from all sides of a story. After watching, reading and listening to countless hours of interviews from the perspective of those who had come to the United States, I came to see the astonishing range of omissions that subjugated the immigrant narrative.

I saw that in mainstream, commercial news, no mention was ever made of the enormous reliance of North American capitalism on migrant labor. It was never explained that families who obtained false social security numbers often ended up paying into the system far more than they could ever take out by way of accessing services (Chomsky 2007). Most importantly, stories never started from the per- spective that those crossing the border were human beings. Rather, the preferred story thought of the aforementioned people as criminals merely breaking laws.

The final question in deconstruction might include:

- How does this information contribute to, create, or reinforce already existing messages that maintain hegemony?

Big businesses largely opposed immigrant rights on the basis of their own self-interest. When people immigrate through legal means, they are afforded the protections of US citizens. This means, for example, that minimum wage laws dictate their hourly pay and that they are entitled to certain basic health benefits depending on the company for which they are working. Many businesses that employ undocumented folks do so because they cannot afford to pay the same number of US citizens a fair hourly wage. The flip side of this maintains that, without illegal immigration, many of these busi- nesses would be unable to sustain themselves without drastic changes in their business models (Chomsky 2007: 37). As such, major institutions (business) supported public policies that contributed to the cultural stigma of undocumented status, even when the covert practices of the same business relied on it to survive. Furthermore, a thorough deconstruction revealed that many of these same companies had engaged in business practices that had greatly weakened economies south of the United States border (Chomsky 1993). This economic instability had driven many who would otherwise be content to stay in their countries of origin to seek work elsewhere, particularly in the United States.

Engage in political struggle in solidarity with the communities I served

I committed myself to keeping an eye out for opportunities from then on that would allow me to expand my consciousness with respect to issues of economic justice and immigrant rights. Several months after my court clinic internship ended, I learned that a local organization was holding a demonstration outside of the ICE detention center on Columbus day. It was not just a sense of frustration and outrage at ICE, but a sense of responsibility as a social worker to improve the community in which I practiced that impelled me to join. The most important thing that I learned early on as a social worker was that I could not treat the individual and ignore the community. To meet my ethical mandate to treat the entire problem, I had to become a clinician activist.

The first rally I attended was put on by a group known as "Resist the Raids," a prominent immigrant rights group in Massachusetts. Resist the Raids featured the voices of many community and thought leaders. Among these was Aviva Chomsky, professor at Salem State University and daughter of prolific anti-imperialist writer Noam Chomsky. The rally was a solidarity march, in that it aimed to show a sense of camaraderie with those who had been most deeply impacted by ICE raids. The route took marchers from the center of a major thoroughfare in Boston to the ICE detention facility known as South Bay Correctional Facility.

A speak-out was held in front of the prison entrance. Families who had lost a loved one to harsh immigration practices told their stories through megaphones with the sound reverberating off of the prison walls. After the speak-out, the contingent of approximately 50 people moved to the other side of the prison, that which faced the windows of jail cells that were currently holding prisoners being detained for immigration-related infractions. During a poignant moment, while we the protesters held up signs in English and Spanish professing solidarity with the prisoners, an inmate pressed his ICE prison uniform against the jail cell window. In synchrony with the protesters outside, who were pounding on drums and railings, he began to pound his fist into the air.

Rescuing the historical memory of change

What followed this rally underlines another part of a liberation health intervention, "rescuing the historical memory [of change]" (Martín-Baró, Aron and Corne 1994: 30). Enticed by the rally and emboldened by the stories of demonstrators whose resistance had a long, rich history I had hitherto been unaware of, I immersed myself in what has been coined "radical history." It was in this search that I found the writing of Dr. Dumont, the psychiatrist who staged a press hearing at the Tobin bridge to publicize Massport exposing the children of Chelsea to harmful lead paint. After I enrolled in a "radical social action" course taught by book editor Dawn Belkin-Martinez, I learned how the Young Lords had taken over Lincoln Hospital to provide detox, or how it was actually the original Black Panther Party under the direction of Huey P. Newton who founded what has become the "Head Start" school breakfast program.

New social workers who look carefully enough will find a bastion of information on radicalism in the field of social work itself. As new students to the field of social work will hopefully learn in introductory policy classes, the field of social work rests on a solid body of sociopolitical activism. Reisch and Andrews (2001) document that Florence Kelley, co-founder of Hull House (one of the vanguard of the settlement house movement) was heavily influenced by the rise of socialism and in regular correspondence with Frederich Engels (p. 18). Unfortunately, this leftist radicalism was largely shut out in a move to legitimize the profession (Reisch and Andrews 2001; Specht and Courtney 1994). Nevertheless, for the past 100 years, some social workers have been combating this deradicalization in much the way described by Zinn or Dumont. In 1976, the NASW code of ethics was amended, to include an ethical mandate to social workers to incorporate the fight for social justice into clinical practice.

I read the late Boston University Professor Howard Zinn, and downloaded lectures he had given on the subjugated narrative of the American labor struggle. I re-educated myself on radical history, and challenged in myself the notion that "no one can fight the system."

As I learned about others before me that had challenged the system, I began to see what Howard Zinn meant (referenced in the beginning of this chapter). While there is a dominant history of domination and subordination, there are other equally important histories of resistance and overcoming oppression. I aligned myself with all who had made a similar commitment. As I continued to move towards a new *subject* role, whereby I had agency and knowledge about the oppressive systems that surround popular social work education, my relationship with "a feeling of unease" (see Figure 2.1) renegotiated. Unease appeared less and less, and when it did, I experienced a sense of agency in defining the problem and consciously choosing my response.

As you will learn in the chapters that follow, liberation health interventions are not uniform. They adhere to the principle that Freire is perhaps most famous for: using the strengths and talents unique to the person or people seeking liberation, and harnessing them in the interest of social change.

I had worked for over a decade prior to graduate school as an information technology consultant, completing tasks such as refurbishing and retrofitting hardware, writing code and maintaining websites. When the opportunity arose to volunteer my skills for groups whose focus was economic justice and immigrant rights, I did not hesitate to re-employ these skills to facilitate electronic communication across activists. What had occupied so much of my adolescence, idling in chat rooms and sharing information, translated beautifully into helping activist communities and underserved communities meet their needs for communications technology. I continue to devote a portion of my time to retrofitting old hardware for donation. As I fill donation requests, this facilitates community and introduces me to circles of which I would otherwise be ignorant. As my world grows wider and diversifies, so too, do the number of different worldviews to which I am exposed.

Not surprisingly, as new horizons open, so too does the need for more self-education, and thus grows the desire to stand in solidarity with the people with whom I come into contact. As Freire stated, liberation is not a thing that is done to a person. It must happen with a person, or more pointedly, a person must liberate themselves (Freire 2000). In such a spirit, a clinician activist is always on the lookout for more ways to raise her own consciousness one struggle at a time.

Reflections

What is described above may colloquially be termed a "radical education." This "radical education" is an essential part of the liberation that is so necessary for social workers entering the field if they wish to engage in liberation health work. Essential to a successful liberation health intervention, as you will see in later chapters, is the ability to bring out relevant historical moments that make an alternate story possible for clients who gain hope from learning about others who have been successful in similar struggles.

For every facet of social life, there is likely to be a matrix of oppression (also known as an *oppressive system*) that influences that facet. And for every matrix of oppression, there are those who have fought this oppression and won. Others are still fighting and many are winning. It is important that clinicians who wish to engage in liberation health work examine the matrices of oppression in the lives of their clients, and engage in active struggle against them. This is what we mean by "activist clinician."

For myself, it was an opportune time to become involved in political activism. On the other side of the world, Egypt and Tunisia were experiencing full-scale rejections of regimes that violated human rights conventions. In the second week of February, Hosni Mubarak, then-President of Egypt, was deposed by non-violent resistance. Around this time in the United States, Scott Walker, then Republican governor of Wisconsin attempted to pass anti-union legislation. Hundreds of thousands of demonstrators occupied the rotunda at the Capital in Madison. A little more than half a year later, Occupy Wall Street took up residence in Zuccotti Park to call attention to the effects of economic imperialism in the United States. Ignacio Martín-Baró would call this the "historical moment," that is to say the unique fingerprint of the state of the world in reference to my understanding of it.

Clinically, I have continued to practice with clients in underserved communities, and have had the privilege of witnessing dozens of personal transformations resulting from this self-same consciousness raising. That is not to say that it has been without difficulty. To be faithful to true liberation requires a degree of intellectual and emotional honesty that does not allow one to escape without examining personal contributions to oppressive matrices. The realization of a clinician's own position in the matrix of power requires a painful truthfulness. Although I am aware of more worlds and ways of being than before my adoption of a clinician activist persona, I must remember that this is not the same as having the experience directly myself. I must confront the reality that try as I can, I will not know involuntary homelessness, hunger or racism. Even were I to choose to live on the streets in solidarity with those most affected by economic imperialism, it would still be by choice. Therefore, clinician activism also requires humility.

As with any clinical practice, continuing education is a part of competence. In the wake of Occupy Wall Street's first year, I have met thousands of people who continue to challenge me and raise my consciousness on a daily basis. Although the push for productivity makes time away from the office difficult, I make sure to carve out time every week for some sort of resistance. This is, in effect, self-care.

In writing this chapter, one theme has resurfaced over and over: I am a very different practitioner now than I was when I began. Although I reflect upon my experiences at the court with some degree of confidence, I felt none of this as a first-time practitioner. With each successive year of practice, I have felt myself become more and more bold about the topics I include in therapy and more radical in the way I understand them. It is with some sadness that I reflect upon what I would have done differently that first year, had I been farther along in this process. I must reconcile, however, that without those first steps, I could not write what I have written above. I encourage readers not to be hard on themselves for finding the application of liberation health to be a difficult process. Challenging dominant worldview is always a difficult task, but I promise that it is worth it.

I hope that the reader will take the aforementioned case presentation and vignette not as an instruction manual, but as inspiration. The work of a liberation health practitioner begins with a fundamental change of perspective, but also a change of heart. Many of us enter into the social work profession buying into the idea that social workers *fix problems*. My hope is that this chapter has altered that idea to represent that social workers *incorporate themselves into solutions*. Perhaps more pointedly, social workers align themselves with clients as they seek the solutions themselves. At the same time, Liberation Health-informed social workers stand side by side with communities in opposing oppression and see this as a vital part of clinical practice.

References

Almeida, R.V., Dolan-Del Vecchio, K., and Parker, L. (2007) Foundation concepts for social justice-based therapy: Critical consciousness, accountability, and empowerment. In E. Aldarondo (ed.), *Advancing Social Justice Through Clinical Practice*. Mahwah, NJ: Lawrence Erlbaum, pp. 175–201.

Capps, R., Castañeda, R.M., Chaudry, A., and Santos, R. (2007) *Paying the Price: The Impact of Immigration Raids on America's Children*. A Report by The Urban Institute. Washington, DC: National Council of La Raza.

Chomsky, A. (2007) *"They Take Our Jobs!" And 20 Other Myths About Immigration*. Boston, MA: Beacon Press.

Chomsky, N. (1993) Notes on NAFTA: "The masters of mankind," *Nation*, 256 (12): 412–16.

Christensen, L. (2012) The classroom to prison pipeline. *Rethinking Schools*, 26 (2): 24–7.

Dean, R. (2004) Looking toward the future in unsettled times. *Smith College Studies in Social Work*, (2004), 74 (4): 579–93.

Dumont, M. P. (1992) *Treating the Poor: A Personal Sojourn Through the Rise and Fall of Community Mental Health*. Belmont, MA: Dymphna.

Dumont, M. P. (1994) *Therapists in the Community: Changing the Conditions that Produce Psychopathology*. Northvale, NJ: J. Aronson.

Freire, P. (2003) *Pedagogy of the Oppressed* (30th anniv. edn.). New York: Continuum International Publishing Group (originally published 1970).

Harro, B. (2000) The cycle of socializations. In M. Adams, W. J. Blumenfeld, R. Castañeda, H. W. Hackman, M. L. Peters and X. Zúñiga (eds), *Readings for Diversity and Social Justice*. New York: Routledge, pp. 15–30.

Kupchik, A. (2010) *Homeroom Security: School Discipline in an Age of Fear*. New York: New York University Press.

Martín-Baró, I., Aron, A., and Corne, S. (1994) *Writings for a Liberation Psychology*. Cambridge, MA: Harvard University Press.

McGoldrick, M. (1998) *Re-visioning Family Therapy: Race, Culture, and Gender in Clinical Practice*. New York: Guilford Press.

McLeigh, J. D. (2010) How do immigration and customs enforcement (ICE) practices affect the mental health of children? *American Journal of Orthopsychiatry*, 80 (1): 96-100.

Minuchin, P., Colapinto, J., and Minuchin, S. (2007) *Working with Families of the Poor* (2nd edn.). New York: Guilford Press.

Reisch, M., and Andrews, J. (2001) *The Road Not Taken: A History of Radical Social Work in the United States*. Philadelphia, PA: Brunner-Routledge.

Reynolds, B. C. (1991) *An Uncharted Journey: Fifty Years of Growth in Social Work* (3rd edn.). Silver Spring, MD: NASW Press.

Specht, H., and Courtney, M. E. (1994) *Unfaithful Angels: How Social Work has Abandoned its Mission*. New York: Free Press.

Zinn, H., and Barsamian, D. (1999) *The Future of History: Interviews with David Barsamian*. Monroe, ME: Common Courage Press.

3

LIBERATION HEALTH AND LGBT COMMUNITIES

Ezekiel Reis Burgin

While this chapter's title uses the acronym "LGBT" (lesbian, gay, bisexual, and transgender people) to encourage recognition, the term that will be used within this chapter is "gender and sexual minority," as it is more encompassing and does not include the negative community history that LGBT does.[1] There is a wide variety of identities that can be considered gender or sexual minorities.[2] All are included, owing to mainstream society's determination that they are outside the bounds of "normal" sexuality and gender.

The language surrounding and used by various gender and sexual minority communities is in flux. As the language continues to change, terms that are considered applicable at the time of printing may no longer be appropriate at the time of reading. As with any marginalized population, it is important to listen to the language that a client uses to describe hirself,[3] and to mirror those terms when working with hir, regardless of terms used in this chapter or elsewhere.

The term "queer" and its history deserve special note. "Queer" has a long history as a slur directed against community members, so its use is controversial; however, it is gaining ground as a politicized and reclaimed umbrella term, especially among younger community members. The term can be a general statement of non-conformity to dominant worldview expectations, a way to push back against hetero-normative cultural expectations. By embracing the "weirdness" of one's gender or sexual orientations, some people, myself included, find community in "queerness."

Given dominant views towards "deviance," some clients may choose to keep their marginalized identities hidden while in public. This presents a clinical hurdle for them: whether and/or when to disclose. Some relatively privileged clients will choose to "out" themselves early in the process, believing that if a clinician cannot accept their marginalized identity at the beginning of the therapeutic process, it will be that much more painful if disclosure happens later. However, for those clients who are multi-marginalized, this may not (appear to) be a tenable option. Their economic resources could make a certain clinic or clinician the only possible option, or their disability or ethnicity could otherwise limit with whom they feel comfortable working. Because of this it is important to treat every client potentially as a gender or sexual minority community member.

Introduction of the author and the institutional context of the case to be presented

The work described in the following case study was carried out at the Rainbow Alliance, a community mental health program in the Pacific Northwest for "LGBTQ" individuals needing day treatment. Clients generally participate for anywhere between two weeks and two months in groups and individual counseling. Dedicated programs such as the Rainbow Alliance are often necessary for many community members, owing to the ways that hetero- and cis-normative[4] spaces can inhibit feelings of "belonging." This author belongs to multiple gender and sexual minority communities. He is young, white, and college educated, with a family history of class privilege. At the time of treatment discussed here, the author was "visibly" trans, as he was usually erroneously perceived by others to be a woman, but introduced himself with male pronouns and a male name. The author was often assigned the cases of trans* clients,[5] often in response to a client's request to have a trans* clinician.

Literature review

Dominant worldview has humans organized by the *gender binary* (Currah, Juang, and Minter 2006; Serano 2007), in which physiological sex, gender, and sexuality are considered set at birth as one of two options: men, who have penises and are attracted to women, and women, who have vaginas and are attracted to men. By our very nature, gender and sexual minority individuals challenge dominant worldviews. *Transgender, transsexual, trans,* and *genderqueer* individuals call into question the assumption that physiological sex and gender are always paired or will remain consistent throughout life; intersex[6] individuals demonstrate that there are no "opposite" sexes (Greenberg 2006), and the existence of *queer,* undecided, lesbian, bisexual, asexual,[7] and gay individuals disputes the idea that all people are attracted to the "opposite" sex.

Typically, *transgender, transsexual,* and *trans* individuals are thought of as identifying as the "opposite" gender (Rudacille 2006; Serano 2007). Some individuals may not feel that their gender aligns with either of the options given in the gender binary. Those individuals may identify as genderqueer (Stryker 2008; Sycamore 2006; Wyss 2004). For genderqueer individuals, *gender-neutral pronouns* can be essential (Stryker 2008; Wyss 2004). Typically, it is best to ask clients what pronouns they prefer be used when speaking about them, regardless of whether you believe they are trans* or not.

Given our societal expectations and cultural assumptions of binary and "normal" sex, therapists using the liberation health model must be prepared to positively affirm the incredible range of normal, healthy human sexuality with clients, despite not knowing if a particular client is a gender or sexual minority. Clients may require help and a "push" towards self-love. Healthy human sexuality is incredibly diverse. Milton Diamond has famously said: "Nature loves diversity. Unfortunately, society hates it" (Rudacille 2006). As clinicians, it is our duty to embrace that diversity.

Oppression and marginalization of gender and sexual minority communities

Gender and sexual minority communities subvert cherished cultural beliefs about how people are meant to be and to love (Greenberg 1988); as such, these populations face prejudice and oppression (Grant, *et al.* 2011; Meyer 2003; Morrow 2001). Violent crime against our communities is common (Federal Bureau of Investigation 2000; Wyss 2004), although it is often under-acknowledged because of prejudice (Amnesty International 2005). Discrimination in employment (e.g. Grant *et al.* 2011; Pizer, Sears, Mallory, and Hunter 2012), healthcare (e.g. Grant *et al.* 2011; Xavier *et al.* 2004), housing (e.g. Ahmed and Hammarstedt 2009; Grant *et al.* 2011; US Department of Housing and Urban Development 2013), and political battles over marriage rights and partnership benefits also contribute to community stress and anxiety (Russell 2000; Russell and Richards, 2003).

The history and present of activism and solidarity in gender and sexual minority communities

Queer and trans* youth are generally not raised by parents in the community, and owing to a dearth of other options, gay bars have historically been important to the process of figuring out what being queer or trans* "means" (Thomas 2011). In the 1960s, raids on gay bars were common across the country, from Los Angeles to New York. The Stonewall Inn was not the first raid which resulted in protests; however, the following protests were the first that garnered national attention (D'Emilio 2002; Duberman 1993). Out of the Stonewall riots arose the modern gay rights movement, with communities galvanized by the realization that change could happen. "It was clear that things were changing. People who had felt oppressed now felt empowered" (Carter 2004: 216–17).

Many of the key players in the Gay Liberation Front (GLF, started after Stonewall) were trans* women of color and bisexual women (Duberman 1993; Stryker 2008), causing the early movement to be intersectionally focused. The GLF was explicitly anti-capitalist and anti-racist, aligning themselves with the Black Panthers. A portion of the UK GLF manifesto lays out how radical they were: "We do not intend to ask for anything. We intend to stand firm and assert our basic rights. If this involves violence, it will not be we who initiate this, but those who attempt to stand in our way to freedom" (Gay Liberation Front 1971).

As queer activists have asserted themselves, medical and mental health communities have been forced to change. In 1986, after decades of activist organizing, the APA removed homosexuality for the second and final time from the revised third edition of its *Diagnostic and Statistical Manual of Mental Disorders* (DSM III). However, the pathologizing of gender and sexual minorities continues into the second decade of the 21st century. Internationally, intersex activists are still struggling to stop the mutilation of intersex infants to conform to expectations of "normal" genitals (Holmes 2006), while trans* activists have lost the most recent fight to get our identities de-pathologized in the fifth edition of the DSM (Fraser, Karasic, Meyer, and Wylie 2010; Serano 2012; Winters 2012a, 2012b).

The mental health professions' views towards gender and sexual minority identities

The APA, together with 12 other organizations, including the National Association of Social Workers, views bisexual, gay, and lesbian sexual orientations as "normal variants of human sexuality" (American Psychological Association 2012: 14), and has publicly denounced so-called "reparative" or "conversion" therapies (Just the Facts Coalition 2008). The APA recommends to psychologists and counselors of bisexual, gay, and lesbian clients that they "understand that lesbian, gay, and bisexual orientations are not mental illnesses" (American Psychological Association 2012: 13). Such guidelines are not in place for working with asexual or trans* clients. Currently, asexual and transgender identities can be, from a DSM diagnostic viewpoint, considered mental illnesses.

The World Professional Association for Transgender Health (WPATH) has recommended that counseling organizations adopt language indicating that gender nonconformity and trans* identities are not inherently mental disorders, and instead, that the psychological *pain* associated with dominant social views regarding gender nonconformity should be considered a treatable mental health concern. However, a distressing number of organizations have yet to follow suit. Too many therapists still advise the equivalent of "conversion therapy" for those who are trans*, suggesting that children who do not identify with their gender-assigned-at-birth should be "taught" to conform (Rosin 2008).

The liberation health model with gender and sexual minority communities

There is a strong theoretical basis for applying a liberatory framework, based on Paulo Freire and Ignacio Martín-Baró's work (see Chapter 1), to gender and sexual minority communities (Russell and Bohan 2007). The liberation health framework revolves around working with marginalized individuals to help to end their oppressions. As members of an oppressed community, gender and sexual minorities benefit from the liberation health model. These communities are also well poised to take advantage of the liberation health model, owing to their history of activism and solidarity.

The literature concerning use of anti-oppressive practice (Hines 2012) and liberation psychology (Moane 2008; Russell and Bohan 2007) with gender and sexual minorities is limited, yet encouraging. The initial and most important step for all liberatory practices is "when the person 'decodes' the messages implicit in the social order" (Hines 2012: 29; Russell and Bohan 2007) and in doing so "grasps the mechanisms of oppression and dehumanization" (Martín-Baró, 1994: 40). Societal homophobia and transphobia can lead to isolation (Beals and Peplau 2005; Szymanski, Chung, and Balsam 2001), self-hatred (Hines 2012; Prilleltensky 2008), and belief in one's inherent sinfulness (Kaufman and Raphael 1996; Tigert 2001). "Decoding" or "deconstructing" these messages allows an oppressed individual the ability to name, and thus combat these cultural forces. Working with community members requires practitioners be willing and able to recognize and then deconstruct cissexist/transphobic[8] and heterosexist/homophobic messages present in our society (Hines 2012; Moane 2008; Russell and Bohan 2007), helping clients to recognize and then combat those messages in their personal lives and on the larger political scale.

In combating oppression, the oppressed also gain the tools needed for greater mental health and self-love. Similar to the feminist movement's mantra that the "personal is political," a liberation framework acknowledges that the personal and cultural are intertwined, and "by changing [our]selves, [we] are altering the sociopolitical world" (Russell and Bohan 2007: 67). In liberation health, both social change and mental wellbeing are the purposes, and simultaneously the means to achieving them.

Case study: "Lucas"

Referral and presenting issue

"Lucas" was a mid-20s Asian-American queer-identified transgender man who presented to the Rainbow Alliance with a diagnosis of depression. His frequent periods of intense suicidality had resulted in seven previous hospitalizations, including one directly prior to his arrival at the program. Lucas was a participant in the program on and off over the course of six months. At intake, Lucas reported self-loathing, flashbacks, insomnia, fatigue, suicidality, trouble trusting others, and anhedonia (at times). He stated that he was "filled up with evil," that he "deserve[d] to suffer," and that "death wouldn't be enough of a punishment" for how "evil" he was.

Current situation

Owing to his hospitalizations and ongoing mental health difficulties, Lucas had been forced to drop out of college and was unable to find and retain a job. In addition, one of the few supportive members of his family had recently died (an aunt), and he had just left inpatient treatment. Lucas's housing situation was unstable during the periods that he attended therapy. When testosterone treatment led to beard growth and voice change, Lucas's parents expelled him from their home, after which he boarded with friends. In groups he was often insightful when choosing to speak, but generally quiet.

Relevant history

Lucas was defined as female at birth and raised as a girl in his family's conservative Christian religious home. He stated that he was anathema to the church, because of being attracted to women (as someone considered to be female), and his status as transgender. Lucas was quite certain that if he were explicitly to tell his family about his gender, it would result in his family believing he was destined for hell. Lucas also sometimes believed this about himself. Lucas wanted to be accepted as part of the faith, and more distressingly for him, wanted to be the type of person who was accepted by the faith. Lucas had at one time attempted to "come out" to his family, only to be told that zie was "possessed by the devil" if zie felt that zie was a man or was attracted to women. Following his aborted coming out attempt, Lucas reported being asked by his mother during a car trip about his sexuality/gender identity. After he lied to his mother, she stated, "Good, because if you had said you were, I would have driven the car off a bridge."

Lucas had a long history of trauma including childhood physical and sexual abuse and assault by an adult family friend (considered an "uncle" to the family) and an older cousin. Family members blamed Lucas for the abuse, and continued to associate with the abusers, requiring that Lucas interact with them in a "respectful" manner. Prior to his most recent suicide attempt, Lucas was sexually assaulted while walking home at night. His family told him "this wouldn't have happened to a real man." He was also not allowed to engage in activities that could have helped him feel safe, (including leaving a light on at night, staying home during family outings where there was a significant risk of being triggered, and avoiding contact with his childhood abusers).

Formulation

On a personal level, Lucas suffered from severe depression, post-traumatic stress disorder (PTSD), and social isolation. Recent life events, including his aunt's death, his sexual assault, and his dismissal from school, combined to increase his stress and his feeling that he was "unlovable."

On a societal level, he was subject to a perfect storm of racism, rape culture, transphobia, sexism, homophobia, ableism, capitalism and productivism.[9] As an Asian-American man, Lucas was subject to racialized images of his gender, namely that Asian-American men are "effeminate." As a survivor of sexual assault and abuse, Lucas was yet again placed into the role of "feminine." These together greatly increased his internalized self-hating narratives about trans* identities, namely that his identity was not genuine or "real." As his own internalized transphobia interacted with these various messages proclaiming his "femininity," he, despite not being a girl, started

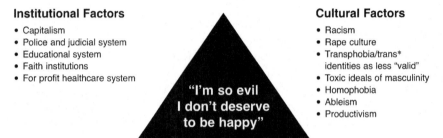

Personal Factors

- Brain chemistry
- Depression
- Loss of loved one
- Social isolation
- Unemployed
- College drop out
- Recent and childhood sexual assaults
- PTSD

Institutional Factors

- Capitalism
- Police and judicial system
- Educational system
- Faith institutions
- For profit healthcare system

Cultural Factors

- Racism
- Rape culture
- Transphobia/trans* identities as less "valid"
- Toxic ideals of masculinity
- Homophobia
- Ableism
- Productivism

"I'm so evil I don't deserve to be happy"

FIGURE 3.1 Liberation health and the LGBT community

Source: Ezekiel Reis Burgin

having to contend with sexist messaging. In his mind, his sexual assault "proved" he was a girl, and his "being a girl" in turn led to his sexual assault. Once Lucas was put on the defensive about his gender, he struggled to assert his masculinity by buying into dominant stereotypes of masculinity. He retreated from exploring emotions with friends, and stopped hugging or acknowledging positive emotions.

Rape culture, together with sexism, homophobia/heterosexism, and trans-phobia, combined to add to his feelings of shame and lack of self-worth. Lucas internalized the cultural messaging that sexual assaults don't happen to "real" men, and that "real" men would (if they somehow did find themselves subject to a sexual assault) respond with anger and violence. Lucas blamed himself for his fear in the face of the assault, as opposed to "wanting to go find the guy and punch him, which all my friends want to do."

Capitalism/productivism and ableism together created an environment that continued to shame Lucas every day. Lucas had been unable to complete college, and because of his depression and PTSD, Lucas was also "unemployable" according to capitalist expectations that workers work the most consistently for the least pay. As he was raised in a productivist/capitalist society, Lucas's understanding of his self-worth was tied to his ability to "produce." As he was unable to "produce" either a college degree or a steady income, Lucas's self-worth was consequently lowered. As his self-worth plummeted, Lucas' ability to maintain expected standards for our capitalist society also decreased, creating a negative spiral of self-hatred.

Institutionally, Lucas was betrayed by the police, the US healthcare system, the education system, and his parents' faith community. The police harmed his sense of self by consistently misgendering him following the assault. At the same time, because of capitalist concerns and lack of universal healthcare, the healthcare systems he entered maintained care only at the minimum level mandated and for the duration paid for by insurance (which likewise attempted to minimize the expense of his treatment). His college also lacked supports for students such as himself. Finally, his family's faith community compounded his oppression and stress, leading him to view himself as "so evil, [he didn't] deserve to be happy."

Applying liberation health: interventions

Owing to the nature of the program and the time frame that Lucas and I had together, my interventions and our work together primarily focused on deconstruction of dominant worldviews. We also worked together to introduce new information into Lucas's conception of self, and ultimately worked to increase Lucas's sense of solidarity.

Deconstructing dominant worldviews

When asked what he felt his problem was, Lucas stated: "I hate myself and I'm evil." In order to fully understand this identified problem, we constructed a liberation health triangle. We constructed our triangle around Lucas's identified problem with points labeled for "personal" issues contributing to his problem, "cultural" issues, and "institutional" issues. As with many clients, Lucas had the greatest ease when attempting to think of "personal" issues contributing to his problem. We discussed his depression, which had a chemical/biological component to it. He also mentioned his lack of friends and familial support, recent family member death, trauma history, unemployment, and inability to finish his college education.

The first step for Lucas in the liberation health model was realizing the power of cultural messages in his own internal experience, to begin "deconstructing the dominant worldview." At first, Lucas was relatively uncertain in naming cultural issues to include in the triangle, but following a few prompts he started to be comfortable acknowledging the systemic cultural assumptions and biases that added to his feelings of shame and "evilness." Together, we named transphobia, racism, homophobia, capitalism, ableism (the view that depression is a "failing"), and individualism, (which holds the myth of self-sufficiency as an ideal).

After Lucas identified systemic oppressions which affected him, we started talking about his own internalized versions of them, where they often came from (including his school, society, and parents' church), and what institutions further bolstered them (including the healthcare industry). Internalized ableism was a very important thread to untangle. Lucas recognized that his self-blame for being "lazy" and lacking in will power was a major factor in his self-hatred, and together we attempted to analyze, and thus combat, these thoughts.

We also talked very carefully around ideas of "sin" and his parents' faith, as much of his internal language centered on evilness. This intervention was delicate, as it was important to note the ways his parents' faith was destructive to his self-identity, without demonizing all religious faith.

Introducing new information

Directly after the sexual assault, it was evident that Lucas needed new information. While he appreciated hearing that his responses to the assault were legitimate, Lucas admitted being unable to fully believe that it was the case. To help Lucas to see himself as part of a larger group of survivors and to get new information about their common experiences, I suggested we call an "LGBTQ" focused domestic violence and sexual assault advocacy and recovery program. At the same time, we discussed getting a trained victim's advocate for future potential interactions with the police. As Lucas did not feel comfortable calling alone, we used the telephone in my office on speakerphone. During the call, Lucas went from listening to me speak, to speaking for himself. He was given information on potential next steps, and was encouraged to follow through.

As Lucas continued to believe on some level that the assaults would not have happened to him if he were a "real" man, we did internet research into resources about sexual assault directed against men. Our search yielded the Rape, Abuse and Incest National Network (RAINN) website, which prompted further contextualization of his symptoms and feelings. Almost all of the psychological effects listed on the website were pertinent to Lucas, but he found it especially validating to see in writing "Psychological outcomes can be severe for men because men are socialized to believe that they are immune to sexual assault and because societal reactions to these assaults can be more isolating" (RAINN, 2009).

After his assaults, Lucas did not feel comfortable expressing weakness or positive emotions, even to friends. This was made evident when other members of his social group showed up for treatment. This group of young men was very physical with each other, jumping on each other's backs and semi-wrestling. However, these displays of physicality were against program rules and distracting for other group members. When called to stop these behaviors, Lucas said these were the only ways he felt comfortable showing affection. "When I punch [him] in the shoulder during group, he knows that means I care about him." He also stated that he and his friends didn't hug, as that would be "weird," and "girly." I introduced the fact that many men *do* feel comfortable expressing their affection, including myself and my friends. We explored together what it would feel like for him to *tell* his friends his feelings, instead of using pseudo-aggression to display them. In discussing this, we also examined ways that men in general are taught not to be kind, and how his own identity as a man who was raised as a girl affects his comfort with expressing positive emotions.

One spur of the moment intervention, after a particularly emotional check-in where Lucas repeated yet again his belief that he wasn't a "real" man, involved my singing a song, along with air guitar, about the inherent "realness" of Lucas' gender identity. This moment of levity allowed Lucas to laugh, and also served as a reminder to Lucas that maleness is not predicated on a specific performance of masculinity, as I was a trans man who was not afraid to make a fool of myself because I knew it made me no less of a man.

Solidarity

Lucas participated in groups while at the Rainbow Alliance. All group members were also community members, and Lucas was able to see a myriad of other relational styles and gender presentations, and to have his own presentation be normalized. Groups also offered Lucas a place to engage in solidarity work around mental illness and trans* and queer identities. When Lucas would report to me that he felt evil, I was able to remind him of the large number of other clients who felt similarly about themselves, and ask him whether he felt *they* were evil. As Lucas was able to see the good in other community members, and to support them in seeing the good in themselves, he grew more comfortable with the idea that he might have some good inside himself as well. Although in our time together he did not get to a place of self-love, Lucas' solidarity with other group members allowed him to entertain the *idea* that he might deserve love.

While at the Rainbow Alliance, Lucas did not have the time or the energy to engage in activism, I encouraged him to start going to local trans* and queer organizing events once his time with the program was over. By the time Lucas left, he had changed from someone who felt he deserved his depression for being "evil" to someone who was able to say he wanted to not be depressed. Lucas has kept in periodic touch with me through the years, and is continuing to engage in solidarity work with local trans* and queer organizations. His depression has not gone, but through activism and community, he is finding increasing strength to love himself and to change the world.

Reflections

While there was not sufficient space in this chapter to fully develop other themes, a chapter with Lucas as a case study could almost as easily have focused on ableism as it did on queer and trans* identities. Writing about Lucas without exploring all of his nuances was very difficult, as his experiences, identities, and oppressions were so very interconnected, intersectional, and integral to his self and to our treatment time and goals. I also was conscious of my desire to have an "LGBT" chapter that did not leave the T "silent" yet again. This urge towards inclusiveness made it difficult to pare Lucas down to a few salient features.

In working at the Rainbow Alliance, I was also confronted with the dichotomy of being a community member and therapist simultaneously. How to balance our professional and personal lives while working in our own communities is a common concern among small town practitioners and those of us working with marginalized populations to which we also belong. In standard psychodynamic theories, it would be my job to keep my personal life from interacting with my professional relationships with clients. As a student, I encountered these beliefs in classes, placement, and with other students. However, queer clinicians have long known that this division is ultimately not possible (Bettinger 2003; Brown 1989; Shernoff 2001). As our communities can be very small, this "professional distance" would require us to forgo activism, and to either minimize friendships and relationships (so as to avoid interacting with former, current, or potential clients), or geographically to remove ourselves, so that our potential community overlap is minimized. This traditional psychodynamic way of looking at therapy inherently privileges those identities that are "normal." Generations of queer clinicians before me have therefore rejected this expectation (Brown 1989). It is because of noting and understanding this failure of certain therapeutic models that I came to liberation health.

In our communities, Lucas's story is all too common. For a therapist who works within these communities, the almost endless examples of discrimination and oppression can too easily become overwhelming. While my more traditional training prepared me to sit and work empathetically with a client while talking about depression, anxiety, or a host of "solely" psychological problems, it did little for my ability to work with a community so steeped in the pain caused by others. The liberation health model has allowed me to work with the Lucases of the world with greater success. If I had not felt "allowed" to connect his struggle with the struggles of others I would easily have felt adrift. Advice that I received from psychodynamically oriented colleagues regarding Lucas was that I needed to learn to sit "neutrally" with Lucas's pain. However, in the fight for social justice and community mental health, there is no such thing as "neutrality" (Hines 2012; Martín-Baró 1994). Allowing Lucas and me to focus on the profound external causes of his pain kept us both from burning out within our therapeutic alliance.

While I hope that this chapter does not scare readers away from working with gender and sexual minority communities, at the same time it is incredibly important to me, for the safety and health of my communities, that those who read this chapter come away with an understanding that these communities need clinicians with true dedication to their concerns. Without sustained effort, clinicians can easily be unaware of common struggles of gender and sexual minority communities, often assuming that the present is much "rosier" than the current reality. This chapter is not, and could not ever be, sufficient for understanding the incredible diversity that is present in gender and sexual minority communities, so in closing, I reiterate: Listen. Listen to the words clients use to describe themselves, listen for how their identities shape their treatment in the outside world, and listen for how they may feel fear and pain due to lack of acceptance. Immerse yourself in the community through blogs, books, comics, movies, and yes, even academic texts. The first intervention you can do as a liberation health clinician is to educate yourself and to continue to educate yourself throughout your life.

Notes

1   It is a common "joke" amongst transgender activists that in the acronyms LGBT and GLBT, "the T is silent" (Greenhouse 2013).
2   A partial list includes asexual, bisexual, gay, genderqueer, intersex, lesbian, queer, questioning/undecided, and trans/transgender/transsexual identities.
3   "Zie," "hir," and "hirself" are one of the most common English gender-neutral pronoun

sets and are used in this chapter for those who identify outside of the gender binary, and to denote hypothetical individuals, being preferable to the incomplete "he or she."

4　"Cis" is a prefix of Latin origin, meaning "on the same side as." In gender studies, it is most often used in the context of "cisgender," a term used to denote an individual who was raised as, and historically was and currently is perceived by others as the same gender they perceive themselves to be. Thus, a space which is "cis-normative" is one which assumes that only cisgender identities are "normal."

5　The term "trans*" is meant to be all-encompassing, using the asterisk as in Boolean searches, denoting a wildcard that could be followed by many things. This term will be used throughout the chapter as an "umbrella term" in order to avoid lengthy (and incomplete) listings of identities.

6　The term "intersex" refers to a wide range of physiological and chromosomal states other than what we think of as "male" and "female." Intersex conditions account for between 0.05 percent and 2 percent of the population (Blackless, *et al.* 2000; Intersex Society of North America 2008; Stryker 2008: 9).

7　While some people may go through periods in their lives where sexual urges are lessened greatly, asexual identified individuals generally feel that their lack of interest in sex is relatively immutable.

8　"Cissexist" refers to the belief that cis* identities are more "authentic" and valuable than trans* identities.

9　The term "productivism" describes the dominant worldview that asserts that people are only worth as much as they "produce" and that only certain things count as "valuable" production. It goes hand in hand with capitalism to make people who are either unable to engage in paid work, or whose work is un/underpaid, feel that their lives and experiences are worth (literally) less.

References

Ahmed, A. and Hammarstedt M. (2009) Detecting discrimination against homosexuals: Evidence from a field experience on the internet. *Economica*, 76 (303): 588–97.

Amnesty International (2005) *Stonewalled: Police Abuse and Misconduct Against Lesbian, Gay, Bisexual and Transgender People in the US.* New York: Amnesty International USA.

American Psychological Association (2012) Guidelines for psychological practice with lesbian, gay, and bisexual clients. *American Psychologist*, 67 (1): 10–42.

Beals, K. P., and Peplau, L. A. (2005) Identity support, identity devaluation, and well-being among lesbians. *Psychology of Women Quarterly*, 29: 140–8.

Bettinger, M. (2003) Sexuality, boundaries, professional ethics, and clinical practice. *Journal of Gay and Lesbian Social Services*, 14 (4): 93–104.

Blackless, M., Charuvastra, A., Derryck, A., Fausto-Sterling, A., Lauzanne, K., and Lee, E. (2000) How sexually dimorphic are we? Review and synthesis. *American Journal of Human Biology*, 12: 151–66.

Brown, L. S. (1989) New voices, new visions: Toward a lesbian/gay paradigm for psychology. *Psychology of Women Quarterly*, 13: 445–58.

Carter, D. (2004) Stonewall: *The Riots That Sparked the Gay Revolution*. New York: St. Martin's Press.

Currah, P., Juang, R. M., and P. Minter, S. (eds) (2006) *Transgender Rights*. Minneapolis, MN: University of Minnesota Press.

D'Emilio, J. (2002) *The World Turned: Essays on Gay History, Politics, and Culture*. Durham, NC: Duke University Press.

Duberman, M. (1993) *Stonewall*. New York: Dutton.

Federal Bureau of Investigation (2000) *Crime in the United States, 1999*. Washington, DC: US Department of Justice.

Fraser, L., Karasic, D., Meyer, W., and Wylie, K. (2010) Recommendations for revision of the

DSM diagnosis of Gender Identity Disorder in adults. *International Journal of Transgenderism*, 12 (2): 80–5.

Gay Liberation Front (1971) Fordham University, Gay Liberation Front: Manifesto London, 1971, revised 1978. Available online at www.fordham.edu/halsall/pwh/glf-london.asp (accessed October 3, 2013).

Grant, J., Mottet, L., Tanis, J., Harrison, J., Herman, J. and Keisling, M. (2011) *Injustice at Every Turn: A Report of the National Transgender Discrimination Survey*. Washington, DC: National Center for Transgender Equality and National Gay and Lesbian Task Force.

Greenberg, D. (1988) *The Construction of Homosexuality*. Chicago, IL: University of Chicago Press.

Greenberg, J. (2006) The roads less traveled: The problem with binary sex categories. In Currah, P., Juang, R. M., and Price Minter, S. (eds) *Transgender Rights*. Minneapolis, MN: University of Minnesota Press, pp. 51–73.

Greenhouse, E. (2013). Dropping the "T": Trans rights in the marriage era. *New Yorker*, April 5. Available online at www.newyorker.com/online/blogs/newsdesk/2013/04/trans gender-rights-gay-marriage-doma.html (accessed October 3, 2013).

Hines, J. (2012) Using an anti-oppressive framework in social work practice with lesbians. *Journal of Gay and Lesbian Social Services*, 24 (1): 23–39.

Holmes, M. (2006) Deciding fate or protecting a developing autonomy? Intersex children and the Colombian Constitutional Court. In Currah, P., Juang, R. M., and Price Minter, S. (eds). *Transgender Rights* (pp. 32–50). Minneapolis, MN: University of Minnesota Press.

Intersex Society of North America (2008) How common is intersex? Available online at www.isna.org/faq/frequency (accessed October 3, 2013).

Just the Facts Coalition. (2008) *Just the Facts About Sexual Orientation and Youth: A Primer for Principals, Educators, and School Personnel*. Washington, DC: American Psychological Association. Available online at www.apa.org/pi/lgbc/publications/justthefacts.html (accessed October 3, 2013).

Kaufman, G., and Raphael, L. (1996) *Coming Out of Shame: Transforming Gay and Lesbian Lives*. New York, NY: Doubleday.

Martín-Baró, I. (1994) *Writings for a Liberation Psychology*. Cambridge, MA: Harvard University Press.

Meyer, I. H. (2003) Prejudice, social stress, and mental health in lesbian, gay, and bisexual populations: Conceptual issues and research evidence. *Psychological Bulletin*, 129 (5): 674–97.

Moane, G. (2008) Building strength through challenging homophobia: Liberation workshops with young and midlife Irish lesbians. *Journal of Gay and Lesbian Social Services*, 20 (1–2): 129–45.

Morrow, D. F. (2001) Older gays and lesbians: Surviving a generation of hate and violence. *Journal of Gay and Lesbian Social Services*, 13 (1/2): 151–69.

Pizer, J., Sears, B., Mallory, C., and Hunter, N. (2012) Evidence of persistent and pervasive workplace discrimination against LGBT people: The need for federal legislation prohibiting discrimination and providing for equal employment benefits. *Loyola of Los Angeles Review*, 45 (3): 715–79.

Prilleltensky, I. (2008) The role of power in wellness, oppression, and liberation: The promise of psychopolitical validity. *Journal of Community Psychology*, 36 (2): 116–36.

RAINN. (2009) Male sexual assault. Rape, Abuse and Incest National Network. Available online at www.rainn.org/get-information/types-of-sexual-assault/male-sexual-assault (accessed October 3, 2013).

Rosin, H. (2008) A boy's life. *The Atlantic*, November 1. Available online at www.theatlantic.com/magazine/archive/2008/11/a-boys-life/307059/1/ (accessed October 3, 2013).

Rudacille, D. (2006) *The Riddle of Gender: Science, Activism, and Transgender Rights*. New York, NY: Anchor Books.

Russell, G. (2000) *Voted Out: The Psychological Consequences of Anti-gay Politics*. New York: New York University Press.

Russell, G. and Bohan, J. (2007) Liberating psychotherapy: Liberation psychology and psychotherapy with LGBT clients. *Journal of Gay and Lesbian Psychotherapy*, 11 (3–4): 59–75.

Russell, G. and Richards, J. (2003) Stressor and resilience factors for lesbians, gay men, and bisexuals confronting antigay politics. *American Journal of Community Psychology*, 31: 313–28.

Serano, J. (2007) *Whipping Girl: A Transsexual Woman on Sexism and The Scapegoating of Femininity*. Berkley, CA: Seal Press.

Serano, J. (2012) Trans people still "disordered" according to latest DSM. Whipping Girl, December 3 [Blog post] Available online at http://juliaserano.blogspot.com/2012/12/trans-people-still-disordered-according.html (accessed October 3, 2013).

Shernoff, M. (2001) Sexuality, boundaries, professional ethics, and clinical practice: Queering the issue. *Journal of Gay and Lesbian Social Services*, 13 (3): 85–91.

Stryker, S. (2008) *Transgender History*. Berkley, CA: Seal Press.

Sycamore, M. (ed.) (2006) *Nobody Passes: Rejecting the Rules of Gender and Conformity*. Emeryville, CA: Seal Press.

Szymanski, D., Chung, B., and Balsam, K. (2001) Psychosocial correlates of internalized homophobia in lesbians. *Measurement and Evaluation in Counseling and Development*, 34: 27–38.

Thomas, J. (2011) The gay bar: Is it dying? *Slate Magazine*, June 27. Available online at www.slate.com/articles/life/the_gay_bar/2011/06/the_gay_bar_6.html (accessed October 3, 2013).

Tigert, L. M. (2001) The power of shame: Lesbian battering as a manifestation of homophobia. *Women and Therapy*, 23 (3): 73–85.

US Department of Housing and Urban Development (2013) *An Estimate of Housing Discrimination Against Same-Sex Couples*. Washington, DC: US Government Printing Office.

Winters, K. (2012a) Third swing: My comments to the APA for a less harmful gender dysphoria category in the DSM-5. *GID Reform Weblog*, June 19. Available online at http://gidreform.wordpress.com/2012/06/19/third-swing-my-comments-to-the-apa-for-a-less-harmful-gender-dysphoria-category-in-the-dsm-5/ (accessed October 3, 2013).

Winters, K. (2012b) An update on gender diagnoses, as the DSM goes to press. *GID Reform Weblog*, December 5. Available online at http://gidreform.wordpress.com/2012/12/05/an-update-on-gender-diagnoses-as-the-dsm-5-goes-to-press/ (accessed October 3, 2013).

Wyss, S. (2004) 'This was my hell': The violence experienced by gender non-conforming youth in US high schools. *International Journal of Qualitative Studies in Education*, 17 (5): 709–30.

Xavier, J., Hitchcock, D., Hollinshead, S., Keisling, M., Lewis, Y., Lombardi, E., Lurie, S., Sanchez, D., Singer, B., Stone, M. R., and Williams, B. (2004) *An Overview of US Trans Health Priorities: A Report by the Eliminating Disparities Working Group*. Washington, DC: National Coalition for LGBT Health. Available online at www.seguridadsocial.ccoo.es/comunes/recursos/99922/504930-Transexualidad__US_Trans_Health_Priorities.pdf (accessed October 3, 2013).

4

WORKING WITH MAJOR MENTAL ILLNESS IN THE COMMUNITY

Chloe Frankel

Introduction

The work described in this chapter took place at a partial hospitalization program (PHP) in an industrial city with a majority of poor, working-class, and immigrant residents. The PHP is a day-treatment option for individuals struggling with mental illness, substance use, or both, who are in crisis but who do not meet level-of-care requirements from insurance companies (i.e., who are not sufficiently dangerous to themselves or others) to qualify for inpatient hospitalization.

Clients are referred to the PHP by outpatient providers, parole officers, emergency room staff, family members, or by self-referral, and participation is voluntary except when court-ordered or mandated by the Department of Children and Families. Services include group and individual therapy, case management, family meetings, and medication consultations with the staff psychiatrist. Services are covered by insurance, and clinicians are required to document client presentation, diagnosis, medication adherence, and progress throughout the course of treatment.

The author was a clinical Master of Social Work intern at the PHP when working on this case. She had learned about liberation health and was encouraged by her professors and supervisor to try applying this theoretical framework. The terms "mental illness" and "homeless" are used to maintain consistency with the language adopted by most social service settings and to reflect the experience of individuals seeking or receiving mental health care. A list of resources, including progressive and radical psychiatry organizations, is included at the end of the chapter.

Client population

Major mental illness is classified as biologically based, chronic or persistent, and with diagnostic features that severely impair a person's cognitive, emotional, social and vocational functioning (SAMHSA 2012). In the past 50 years, four events have produced drastic changes in the understanding, diagnosis, and treatment of major mental illness: deinstitutionalization, the emergence of anti-psychotic medications, the patients' rights movements since the 1960s, and cuts to social services including mental health treatment, public housing, job training programs, cash assistance, and community services (Lamb 2001).

In the 1950s and 1960s, public critiques of living conditions in state mental hospitals, the rise of anti-psychotic medication, and advocacy for more community-based services created a backlash against long-term institutionalization. Deinstitutionalization dramatically reduced the number of people in long-term care facilities; however, the process was plagued by poor implementation, fragmented social services, and funding deficits (Lamb 2001). The release of many formerly institutionalized individuals coincided with cuts to the very services needed to support them. In the context of an economic recession and increased military spending post-2001, States continue to face pressure to cut back on allocations for public programs, including those related to mental illness (Bazelon Center for Mental Health Law 2011).

A lack of political will and financial commitment to mental healthcare has taken a toll on the indigent mentally ill. In Massachusetts, for example, budget cuts of nearly US$85 million to the Department of Mental Health (DMH) have been associated with understaffing and unsafe working conditions for counselors, unmanageably high caseloads, the closing of rehabilitation and job-training programs, and the loss of nearly 500 inpatient psychiatric hospital beds (Applebaum and Healy 2011). A common strategy in budget negotiations is to cut one type of service (e.g., emergency care) to free up money for another (e.g., long-term community support), but this approach is self-defeating, as it leaves clients continually vulnerable. The DMH Task Force on Safety states: "enhancing some services by diminishing others only moves risks from one place to another" (Applebaum and Healy 2011: 6).

Inadequate psychiatric resources have pushed the burden of caring for the mentally ill onto systems not well equipped to do so, like the criminal justice system (French 1987). Arrest and incarceration of the mentally ill, even for minor infractions, carries long-term damaging consequences. These may include being denied the right to vote, losing eligibility for public housing, and facing limited employment opportunities. In other words, criminal justice involvement further cuts individuals off from the services they need to live in the community. Public housing has a "one strike" policy, in which any infraction can result in permanent eviction. This guarantees homelessness for many individuals with a mental illness (Sun 2012) and feeds into a cycle of poverty, making it harder to establish permanent housing and employment, and more likely that arrest and incarceration will re-occur (Lamb 2001).

According to the National Homeless Coalition (NCH 2006), 20–25 percent of the homeless population in the United States suffers from some form of severe mental illness. Street living comes with attendant risks of random violence, theft, sexual assault, extreme weather conditions, police harassment and brutality, a lack of personal safety, and high stress levels. The impact of traumatic experiences is well-documented among homeless mentally ill persons (Earley 2006; Kim, Ford, Howard, and Bradford 2010; Perron, Alexander-Eitzman, Gillespie, and Pollio 2008) and is associated with decompensation, instability, and more acute and frequent psychotic symptoms. Additionally, mentally ill individuals are more than three times as likely to have a co-occurring substance abuse disorder than adults without a mental illness (SAMHSA 2012). Addiction is discussed more thoroughly in Chapter 6.

The victimization of mentally ill individuals through institutionalization and discrimination gave rise to several advocacy groups and legislative changes in the late 20th century, including the formation of the National Alliance for Mental Illness (NAMI) and the passage of the Americans with Disabilities Act in 1990. NAMI and other groups raise awareness of mental illness, secure resources for research and treatment, fight discrimination, and provide support and solidarity to mentally ill individuals and their friends and families.

Although significant battles have been fought over the rights of mental health patients to make decisions regarding their own care (Sullivan 1992), the reality of a managed care system means they have little say when it comes to the length or types of treatment available to them. The current landscape of social services reflects the damages incurred by poor funding, pressure from insurance companies to cut costs, and an increasing trend towards privatization. The result is a web of poorly connected and inefficient programs, lacking the consistency and continuity of care that would offer the best hope for stability (Lamb 2001). An absence of universal health coverage, along with reliance on public insurance and assistance programs, leaves the lives of mentally ill persons particularly susceptible to disruption as a result of public policy. For this reason, mental health clients should especially be engaged in discussions of healthcare, budget decisions, and social service policies.

Literature review

Much of the current literature on major mental illness emphasizes biological and intrapersonal explanations and solutions. Many treatment approaches focus on behavior modification, medication compliance, and case management to help clients navigate a fragmented social service system (Sun 2012). These approaches reinforce a belief that mental illness is an individual problem, and that improvement depends on the will power, behavior changes, and decisions of mentally ill persons.

In contrast, a liberation health approach places individual experience within a context of social, political, economic, and institutional factors; biological and intrapersonal elements are one part of the whole picture. In developing a liberation health practice with mental health clients, I drew on the following concepts and historical references: raising critical consciousness (Freire 1970), de-ideologizing everyday experience (Martín-Baró, Aron, and Corne 1994), and the anti-psychiatry and patients' rights movements (Aldarondo 2007; Laing 1969; Szasz 1977).

Central to liberation health is Freire's (1970) concept of *conscientizacao* (usually translated as conscientization or critical consciousness), defined as "learning to perceive social, political, and economic contradictions, and to take action against oppressive elements of reality" (p. 35). With mental health clients, raising critical consciousness might include a discussion about the factors that contribute to poor mental health, such as the unavailability of adequate housing, health care, employment opportunities, and community support. Clinicians need not have pre-existing knowledge of these issues; rather the clinician and client together will be "co-investigators" (Freire 1970: 81) who jointly increase their critical consciousness through dialogue with one another (Almeida, Dolan-Del, and Parker 2008).

Martín-Baró, *et al.*'s (1994) model of "de-ideologizing everyday experience" (p. 31) builds on Freire's assertion that effective work with the oppressed must stem from their understanding of their own lived experience. As will be discussed later, useful exercises include those that explore daily life with a mental illness, issues of stigma, and debunking stories and assumptions surrounding mental illness in popular culture. These joint explorations, based on a client's personal experience, help soften internalized stereotyping and self-reproach, connect individuals to a sense of solidarity with others, and mobilize people to seek justice and improve society.

Another important body of work is the writing and activism of current and ex-patients and professionals within and outside of the field of psychiatry. Originators of the anti-psychiatry movement, starting with Foucault (1988), considered psychiatric diagnosis a tool for social control and questioned its motives and legitimacy. Szasz (1977), Goffman (1970), and others objected to involuntary commitment, forced treatment, and over-medication of the mentally ill, which they viewed as a means to intimidate, detain, or control patients. Breggin (1991) and Ginsberg (2006) raised concerns about harmful effects of psychotropic medications and the impact of psycho-pharmaceutical companies on research and treatment. Claude Steiner, founder of Radical Psychiatry, purported that "all functional psychiatric difficulties are forms of alienation resulting from the mystified oppression of people who are isolated from each other" (Corsini 1981: 724), and Marxist psycho-analyst David Cooper (1971) saw revolutionary potential in "madness," which he framed as a method for individuals and groups to make themselves "ungoverned and ungovernable" (p. 97).

The views of anti-psychiatry and consumer-rights advocates are controversial, particularly those who would eschew all medication; however, they offer a useful stance for theorizing issues related to mental health. In general, anti-psychiatrists favor peer-to-peer treatment and recovery models that operate with patient consent in non-restrictive, calming and peaceful environments (Laing 1969). Rather than view mental health symptoms as pathological, activists and advocates embrace a wider range of social behaviors and thought, and they espouse the notion that society itself, and not the individual, might be maladjusted (Laing, 1969; Foucault 1988; Szasz 1977). These values inform liberation health work: emphasis on patients' rights and self-determination, the use of humane and least restrictive forms of treatment, and the inclusion of clients and their family members in treatment decisions.

Liberation health offers opportunities to make the process of treatment more egalitarian and empowering for clients and therapists alike. The combination of reflection and action, what Freire and Martín-Baró both call "praxis," demands joint accountability from the client and clinician to not only name injustice, but to take corrective action against it. Liberation health practice, which emphasizes the clinician's and the client's roles in changing society, offers opportunities for oppressed individuals to feel powerful, resourceful, and influential when standing in solidarity with their allies and peers.

Case summary

Referral and presenting issue

Ana is a 33-year-old Latina of Puerto Rican descent who became homeless following the death of her mother, who was ill with multiple sclerosis and passed away three months prior to Ana's admission to the PHP. Ana was referred to the PHP by a caseworker at her homeless shelter who became concerned when Ana stopped taking her medication and talked about wanting to end her life. Ana is single, with no children, and has no family in Massachusetts. She has a diagnosis of bipolar II disorder, for which she takes a mood-stabilizing medication.

Relevant history

Ana is the youngest of three children, with one full brother and a half-sister from her mother's first marriage. Both of her parents were alcoholics and her father left the family when Ana was young. Her mother had multiple sclerosis and was very ill throughout Ana's life; she was eventually unable to walk and required home care. Owing to their mother's illness, Ana and her brother were raised by their older half-sister. When she was 14, Ana and her siblings moved to Florida, where she completed high school and attended community college. She describes herself as a "good girl" who worked hard in school and was eager to please her teachers and older sister. She was very close with her sister, whom she described as her "protector." However, Ana often felt like the "odd one out" in her family, and reports that her brother, aunts and uncles, and many cousins made fun of her.

Ana struggled with depression for much of her life, but it got worse in college where she had few friends and felt like she didn't fit in. Towards the end of college, Ana had her first manic episode, during which she slept for only two hours a night, began writing a memoir, and left school to move with a boyfriend to Virginia, where she had a series of jobs and was fired for "personal difficulties" and "getting in fights" with her bosses and other staff members. After a year, Ana's boyfriend broke up with her and she moved back to Florida to be near her family. Her older sister insisted that Ana be seen for a psychiatric evaluation. She was diagnosed with bipolar disorder, and began taking medication to stabilize her mood. Ana then had several years of stability, during which she completed her bachelor's degree, got a job in retail, and lived in an apartment with her sister.

In 2009, Ana's sister died suddenly of a brain aneurysm. This had a profound impact on Ana, who is "still dealing with the grief." Shortly after her sister's death, Ana moved to Massachusetts to care for her mother, who had moved there to have access to better healthcare. Ana spent two years living in her mother's apartment and was unable to work during this period because of the demands of caring for her mother. After her mother passed away, Ana had to vacate the apartment because her name was not on the lease. She was unemployed, homeless, and on a four-year waiting list for public housing.

Current situation

Ana's older brother lives with his wife and children in Puerto Rico in the family's home (inherited from their mother), which Ana feels is unfair. Her brother sends her a small amount of money every month, but has made no offer to help her find housing or return to Puerto Rico. Ana believes that he is ashamed of her and that he sees her as irresponsible and incompetent because of her mental illness. She has talked about returning to Puerto Rico, but feels that it is important to live "on her own" and learn to be "independent from [my] family." She expresses ambivalence about getting help from her family because she feels stigmatized and infantilized by them.

Formulation

Ana is a 33-year-old Puerto Rican woman referred to the PHP after going off her medication and expressing suicidal ideation at the homeless shelter where she was staying. Ana is unemployed, homeless, and has a diagnosis of bipolar II disorder. Her

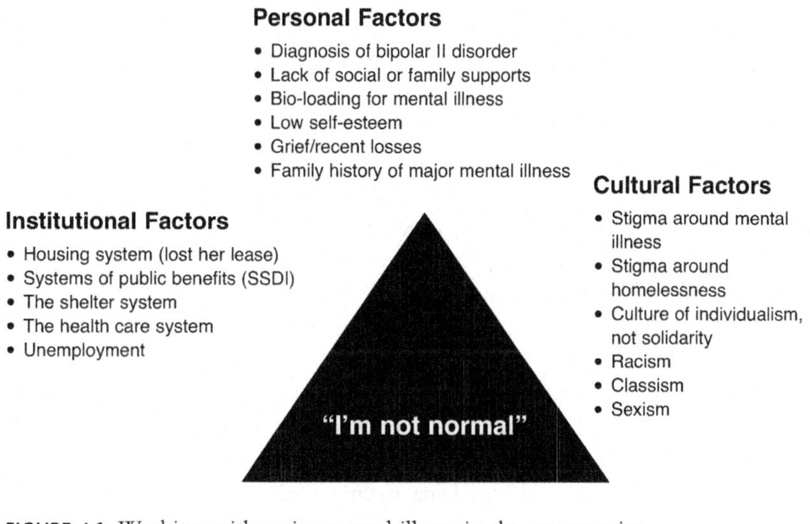

Personal Factors
- Diagnosis of bipolar II disorder
- Lack of social or family supports
- Bio-loading for mental illness
- Low self-esteem
- Grief/recent losses
- Family history of major mental illness

Cultural Factors
- Stigma around mental illness
- Stigma around homelessness
- Culture of individualism, not solidarity
- Racism
- Classism
- Sexism

Institutional Factors
- Housing system (lost her lease)
- Systems of public benefits (SSDI)
- The shelter system
- The health care system
- Unemployment

"I'm not normal"

FIGURE 4.1 Working with major mental illness in the community
Source: Chloe Frankel

understanding of her own situation is that she has had "bad luck" and often been a "victim." She perceives herself as someone with a mental illness, though she feels embarrassed about being labeled as such. For instance, although her medication helps with her depression, she says she is embarrassed to be taking it because it proves that she is "crazy." She feels disappointed by how her life has turned out and is especially troubled by the idea that she is not "normal," which for her would mean having a job, a home, a husband, and children.

Personal factors

Ana's diagnosis of bipolar II disorder is significant, owing to the cycling of her moods and periods of instability when she is either manic or very depressed. In the context of life stressors that would be challenging for anyone, the loss of a sister and mother; frequent moving; job loss and unemployment; homelessness, Ana's mood fluctuations are an added element of stress. They have made her particularly susceptible to feeling incapacitated by grief or depression, or to making impulsive decisions during manic episodes. This has made it difficult for her to hold down a job, maintain relationships, or develop long-term stability.

Cultural factors

Ana's self-description indicates the degree to which she had internalized messages about mental illness that are pervasive in society. As Stefan describes, discrimination against mental illness contributes to a self-fulfilling prophecy:

> Discrimination can cause disability; it is like an infection striking an already vulnerable and struggling soul. When the person who was thrown out of school or denied a job breaks down, the discriminatory prophecy fulfills itself. The connection between the discrimination and the breakdown is lost.
>
> (Stefan 2001: xiii)

Ana felt trapped by this "discriminatory prophecy" in both family and employment contexts. When she lost jobs or had to get treatment for her depression or mania, her bosses and family members viewed this as evidence of her incompetence and inability to function on her own. No one stopped to consider how job loss or family judgment may have contributed to her depression and low self-esteem in the first place.

Mental illness discrimination is often compounded by racial, gender, and cultural stereotypes:

> women who are considered mentally ill are considered much less able to care for themselves and much less likely to be competent; minority employees with disabilities are deemed lazy malingerers trying to take advantage of the system for 'extra benefits,' and so on.
>
> (Stefan 2001: 10)

As the sole living daughter, Ana was expected to be a personal caretaker for her mother, though she was simultaneously considered too incompetent to care for herself. Her brother in Puerto Rico contributed financially and assumed legal guardianship of their mother. Ana therefore had no decision-making power, despite being the one who physically cared for her mother on a daily basis. Meanwhile, she felt that the disability and Medicaid workers treated her and her mother with disdain, and they once accused Ana's mother of exaggerating her illness so that she could collect and send money back to Puerto Rico.

Ana also faced classism because of her employment status, finding it harder and harder to return to the workforce once she had been out of work for a while. She reflected this shame in her own assertion that there was something "wrong" with her for not having a job despite her previous educational and vocational achievements. Missing from this interpretation was an analysis of what her options had been: she faced an impossible dilemma of choosing between a job or supporting a sick family member. Though Ana's employment history had been spotty, she may have had more success had she been granted the time and resources to devote to stabilizing her own mental health and reaping the rewards of longer-term employment (including health benefits, retirement savings, etc.). Although Ana was able to maintain a home and pay the bills with her mother's disability checks, there was no safety net for her when those payments stopped.

Finally, while caring for her mother, Ana was socially isolated. Other family members lived far away and were not available to provide day-to-day support, and she had limited opportunities or finances to socialize. Over time, Ana came to feel increasingly isolated and depressed managing a difficult situation on her own. This isolation continued when Ana became homeless. Her family members were ashamed of her, and there existed even within the homeless community an attitude of "every woman for herself" and a culture of distrust due to the frequency of thefts in the shelters.

Institutional factors

Multiple institutional factors affected Ana's situation. Ana and her mother were dependent on Medicaid and social security for their livelihood, but Ana found the system of public benefits confusing and inaccessible. For the first year as a caretaker for her mother, she had no income and shared her mother's disability check. Eventually, Ana learned about a program in Massachusetts allowing family caretakers to earn some money from the federal government, and she applied. After a three-month process she was approved, but she only received the checks for seven months before her mother passed away and all payments stopped.

Another institutional element that greatly impacted Ana's care was the healthcare system. In addition to her mother's illness, Ana had her own physical and mental health issues. One of the reasons that she stayed in Massachusetts (rather than returning to Puerto Rico or moving in with cousins or family members in other states) was that her health benefits were better in Massachusetts than in any other state. She was able to get healthcare that was potentially life-saving, but it left her isolated and depressed.

The housing system in the United States also played an important role. Once Ana's income disappeared, she became homeless almost immediately. The overloaded public housing system was quick to evict Ana after her mother passed away. With no savings and no family who could take her in, Ana found herself with no options other than homeless shelters or living on the street. Homelessness in the United States is, for many people, only a paycheck or a medical emergency away.

Once Ana became homeless, she had to navigate the shelter system. While Massachusetts has some long-term shelter and transitional living programs, these are exclusively designated for families (mainly women with children), victims of domestic violence, and/or individuals with substance use issues. Single adults are directed to a handful of short-term shelters that offer beds for only a few consecutive nights at a time. In some cases, a bed is not guaranteed and individuals must participate in a daily lottery for beds each night. On any given afternoon, Ana was not sure where she would be sleeping that night.

Given the circumstances, it was nearly impossible for her to establish a routine. Just as she began to settle in and develop relationships with staff and fellow residents, she would have to move. She kept her belongings (including her psychopharmaceutical medications) in a suitcase and had to be ready to change locations at a moment's notice. She had to take different bus routes every day to get from the shelter where she was staying to her appointments. Ana was well organized, but the frequent moving took its toll, and she was often exhausted. Although Ana was looking for work, this setup was not conducive to applying for jobs.

The shelter system, with its strict rules and guidelines, can also be infantilizing. Ana liked to go to the library, but was denied a bus pass to get there, leaving her with nothing to do during the day. She felt belittled by the staff, and struggled to advocate for herself when, for instance, a staff member mixed up her medications with those of another resident. Ana was fearful of speaking up about this mistake because she didn't want to "get in trouble." This fear was grounded in the fact that Ana could be banned from a shelter if she got into an argument with staff members, and this would further limit her options of where to stay.

Interventions

Ana's and my work together utilized one-on-one meetings, group therapy sessions, and resources and advocacy efforts in the community at large. We identified three primary foci for our work together: the first was to develop critical consciousness (Freire 1970; Martín-Baró, et al. 1994; Almeida, et. al. 2008) about the experience of homelessness and major mental illness, and to deconstruct dominant worldview messages about these issues. The second was to develop an action plan that included building a support system and identifying employment and housing opportunities for Ana. The third and final intervention called on both me and Ana to broaden the scope of our work outside of the clinical setting and to engage in educational and advocacy efforts related to the needs of homeless mentally ill persons in Boston and beyond.

Part I: The triangle

During Ana's initial assessment, she tended to personalize her problems and viewed them through the narrow lens of her "downward spiral" towards homelessness. By engaging in an analysis of her problems that took cultural and institutional factors into account, Ana became less invested in a self-critical way of viewing her situation. The Freirean analysis helped Ana see how political and social institutions had contributed to a no-win situation for her.

The triangle shed light on some aspects of Ana's situation that were "not her fault." For instance, since Massachusetts does not provide personal caretakers of sick family members with a living wage, Ana was forced to live in poverty. She would have had to work and pay for homecare for her mother, or, as she chose to do, stay home from work and care for her mother herself. The cultural expectations and pressure on women to be caretakers also took its toll, leaving Ana resentful of her role as her mother's caretaker but also guilt-ridden about not being able to do more. Finally, the scarcity of available public housing in Boston contributed to Ana's eviction and to the lack of housing options she faced afterward. Seeing all this, Ana became less invested in a self-blaming analysis of her situation, and her depression began to lift.

Part II: Deconstructing myths and stereotypes

Ana tended to view her mental health diagnosis and homelessness as personal problems that her family and friends could not understand. Additionally, she was judgmental about other mentally ill and homeless people. By challenging Ana's preconceived notions, I encouraged her to think about homeless mentally ill people as a group subjected to a specific set of social policies and biases.

During one of our sessions, Ana and I made a list of all the myths and stereotypes about mental illness and homelessness in American culture. These included things like "having a mental illness means you're not like other people"; "all homeless people are drug addicts"; "mentally ill people can't have jobs"; "homeless people are dirty"; "homeless people are crazy"; and "it's not 'normal' to be homeless and to have a mental illness." I asked Ana to re-examine these myths and stereotypes in the context of her own experience with mental illness and being homeless. She was able to identify several people, herself included, who proved these stereotypes wrong. As we talked more about what it feels like to have a mental illness and how people become homeless, she developed a more complex view of the factors that lead to mental illness and homelessness. Thinking about people she had met in the shelter, Ana identified factors that had made their situations more difficult such as lack of access to treatment facilities, premature endings of treatment due to insurance cut-offs, a lack of community support, and difficulties finding employment owing to stigma and discrimination.

As Ana developed a more nuanced understanding of mental illness and homelessness, she began to express a greater sense of solidarity with other homeless people with mental illness diagnoses. She made friends with several women in the shelters, and together they began to look out for each other, give each other small gifts and tokens of friendship, and build a small community within the shelter. This progress was significant because it was a rebuttal against the internal divisiveness that so often plagues stigmatized groups. By finding a sense of solidarity within the homeless community, Ana gathered strength to manage her grief and depression, and she also became more comfortable speaking up about the unfair treatment she occasionally received in the shelters. For instance, Ana successfully advocated for herself and was able to get a bus pass to go to the library. This enabled her to begin looking for a job, and she began to discuss her plans for getting out of the shelter, though, significantly, she also spoke about the importance of her friends from the shelter and her plan to keep in contact with them.

Part III: Identifying injustice and taking action

In group therapy sessions, Ana spoke about her frustration towards her brother and sister-in-law. She expressed anger and hopelessness about her relationship with them, and felt helpless to advocate for herself and the inheritance that she was owed. With this issue, I used a theatrical approach to bring the voices of her brother and sister-in-law into the room. I asked other group members to role-play Ana's brother and sister-in-law, and I asked a third group member to act out the part of Ana herself. Ana was then put in the role of director, describing the situation and instructing the actors in the scene. This structure allowed Ana to see her situation from an outsider's perspective, and to gain a more objective point of view.

The scene that unfolded included a conversation between Ana and her brother and sister-in-law in which she was able to challenge them about not sharing the family inheritance with her and explain her feelings of abandonment and rejection. The actors in the scene described their own grief and sorrow over the deaths of Ana's mother and older sister. They expressed affection for Ana, along with their concerns and worries about her ability to manage money by herself or to live independently. They spoke about wanting to support her, but not being sure of what she most needed or wanted. They also described their own financial and personal struggles, which led them to feel proprietary over the family inheritance.

After the scene was over, Ana described feeling much more sympathetic and understanding towards her brother and sister-in-law. She was particularly moved to hear that they shared in her grief over the loss of her mother and sister. Other group members shared their own stories of navigating family relationships and trying to stand their ground in disagreements. These stories helped reinforce that Ana was not alone in her struggles to establish healthy and respectful relationships with her family. There was a sense of solidarity among group members who had also faced discrimination or poor treatment from family as a result of their mental health diagnoses. They were able to brainstorm and offer useful suggestions about how to negotiate with family members.

Ana recognized that her unstable employment history and impulsive behavior did create valid reasons for her brother and sister-in-law to have concerns about her ability to manage money and maintain employment. In response to this, she agreed to work closely with a case manager at her shelter to find proper outpatient treatment, to set up a bank account that she would allow her brother to monitor, and to seek supportive employment. As a final step in this part of the intervention, I referred her to a legal aid program that would help her review her mother's will and redistribute the inheritance that she was owed.

Part IV: Tying into the bigger picture and the larger struggle

After two weeks, my work with Ana was cut short when her insurance company deemed her "stable" enough to leave the partial hospitalization program. Despite our termination, I consider a final element of my work with Ana to be my own education and immersion in the homeless community of Boston. Simultaneous to Ana's admission at the partial program, Occupy Boston was beginning to take hold in the city's financial district. The Occupy movement attracted many people who live on the streets, many of them with mental health diagnoses. The movement was built on the premises of re-claiming and living in public spaces, airing grievances about wealth disparities, and giving voice to the "99 percent" of Americans demanding better housing, healthcare, education and jobs.

The most important avenue to understanding and being able to effectively work with homeless and mentally ill clients was to join with them outside of clinical settings, in the spaces that they occupy in the world. Being part of Occupy was a step in this direction. I learned about life in public places and was engaged in negotiations with the police as well as the challenges of living on the street (including finding food, bathrooms, and water). This experience helped me better understand my homeless comrades and those with mental illnesses when I joined my voice with theirs in demanding basic needs and justice: food, clothing, a means of communication, safety, and freedom of movement, access, and self-determination.

Reflections

My experience practicing liberation health as an intern at a PHP raised important questions related to my professional identity, my work with clients, and my orientation as a clinician activist. In this section, I will discuss how it impacted my work with Ana and changed me as a clinician.

Like most mental health service agencies, the PHP depends financially on a managed care health system in which cost effectiveness and evidence-based practice are paramount. Insurance stipulations direct treatment towards short-term stabilization with a focus on measurable behavior change. The goal of treatment is not to change the world, but to help clients through a period of crisis and get them stable enough to function in their communities. In this context, it is considered naïve at best, and dangerous at worst, to introduce ideas or questions that challenge the status quo, and to invite clients to be more active, vocal, and even critical of the mental health care and social service systems.

Practicing liberation health therefore felt risky to me. It is one thing to recognize that mental illness diagnoses are stigmatizing; it is another to raise a question in staff meetings about whether a client fully understands and agrees with his or her diagnosis. From my liberation health colleagues, mentors, and the authors whose work informed this book, I drew strength and courage to ask problem-posing questions, to look for opportunities to enhance critical consciousness, and to identify explicitly as a clinician activist. Yet I feared repercussions: everything from having my comments and questions in staff meetings be ignored or dismissed to having management reprimand me or limit my caseload. As an intern, I often framed my questions in terms of my own curiosity and learning, and this gave me some leeway. Employees, however, face greater pressure, both implicit and explicit, to abide by the procedural guidelines and values of their host institution.

The culture that discouraged socio-political discussion was subtle but pervasive. I noticed that other social workers repeatedly disengaged when a question arose about the availability of resources for housing, treatment, or public benefits. There existed among the staff as well as among many clients a sense of defeatism and a belief that funding for public services and health care was a fixed reality, that the process of social protest was too time-consuming and ineffective, and that the best course of action was to adapt to scarcity. Activism or organizing in the community was dismissed as non-clinical and outside the purview of the social workers' roles. Indeed, my own involvement in Occupy Boston was conducted on my own time, and would not have been considered part of my "clinical hours."

I hesitated to discuss Occupy Boston with Ana. I feared that this would distract or detract from our work together, and questions of "clinical appropriateness" that had been imparted to me in graduate school rang through my head: *Is it relevant to the therapeutic concerns of the clients? Does discussion of those issues stem from the client's expression of interest, or is the therapist pushing his or her own political agenda?* Ultimately I realized that, while framed as a protection of clients' rights, these questions are rife with contradiction. For example, where is the concern for clients' rights when it comes to labeling individuals with a stigmatizing diagnosis without their consent, prescribing psychotropic medications, or pushing clients to engage in certain kinds of intrusive treatments like electro-convulsive therapy?

Certainly a responsible clinician should assess a client's openness to and interest in discussing socio-political issues, and should proceed accordingly. Some clients may be hesitant to discuss socio-political issues, fearing repercussions, or may try to abide by what they think they are "supposed to" talk about in therapy. However, I found that when I did open the door to socio-political discussion with clients, they were often many steps ahead of me. Anyone who had been in and out of the mental health, drug treatment, criminal justice, or shelter system, or had received public benefits, generally had a much more thorough and nuanced understanding of these systems than I did, with opinions to match. As a liberation health clinician, I was able to affirm for my clients, rather than deny, that there were instances of mistreatment, injustice, and skewed societal values that had contributed to their personal struggles. I focused on helping clients tease out the various threads of discrimination and self-blame that kept them feeling stuck, helpless, or depressed, and channel their existing knowledge and frustration about socio-political realities into avenues for action.

A final question is whether Liberation Health is notably different or offers benefits lacking from other therapeutic interventions. When Ana left the Partial Hospitalization Program she was less depressed, no longer expressing suicidal thoughts, felt more empowered and connected to others, and had a follow-up plan to address her family and financial struggles. These outcomes were achieved through a variety of interventions including medication, group therapy, and case management. However, the liberation health approach is distinctive as a set of principles: it privileges the needs of those being served by mental health institutions over the needs of those providing service; it views social structures as malleable; and it encourages self-determination and collective advocacy for justice.

Liberation health calls for a model of mental health work that asks not just how individuals can better adapt to their world, but how our world can better adapt to its individuals and communities, and, in so doing, perhaps become a more compassionate and just place. This requires collective action, accountability, and the willingness to hold complex truths in our minds and hearts simultaneously. As Martín-Baró, *et al.* (1994), in writing his prescription for liberation psychology, said: "Our imperative is to examine not only what we are but also what we might have been and, above all, what we ought to be, given the needs of our people" (p. 38).

Addendum

In late 2012, Ana transitioned out of temporary shelter and moved into a permanent residence house with her own room and housemates who are "like family." In December, she helped prepare and serve holiday meals, which "create[d] a great sense of community in the house," she says. She is participating in a workforce re-entry program and looks forward to eventually moving into a "little apartment" of her own.

Resources

Crooked Beauty (film by Ken Paul Rosenthal): "A poetic documentary that chronicles artist activist Jacks McNamara's transformative journey from childhood abuse to psych ward inpatient to pioneering mental health advocacy. It is an intimate portrait of her intense personal quest to live with courage and dignity, and a powerful critique of standard psychiatric treatments." Available online at www.crookedbeauty.com (accessed October 3, 2013).

The Icarus Project: "A radical mental health support network, online community, and alternative media project by and for people struggling with extreme emotional distress that often gets labeled as mental illness." Available online at http://theicarusproject.net/ (accessed October 3, 2013).

National Alliance on Mental Illness: "The nation's largest grassroots mental health organization dedicated to building better lives for the millions of Americans affected by mental illness. NAMI advocates for access to services, treatment, supports and research and is steadfast in its commitment to raise awareness and build a community for hope for all of those in need." Available online at www.nami.org (accessed October 3, 2013).

MindFreedom International: www.mindfreedom.org
Disability Rights International: www.disabilityrightsintl.org
National Empowerment Center: www.power2u.org
Radical Psychology Network: www.radpsynet.org
National Paranoia Network: www.nationalparanoianetwork.org
World Network of Users and Survivors of Psychiatry: www.wnusp.net
Mad Pride: http://en.wikipedia.org/wiki/Mad_Pride
Soteria: http://en.wikipedia.org/wiki/Soteria

References

Aldarondo, E. (ed.) (2007) *Advancing Social Justice Through Clinical Practice*. Mahwah, NJ: Lawrence Erlbaum.

Almeida, R. V., Dolan-Del, V. K., and Parker, L. (2008) *Transformative Family Therapy: Just Families in a Just Society*. Boston, MA: Pearson/Allyn and Bacon.

Applebaum, K. L. and Healy, P. F. (2011) Report of the Massachusetts Department of Mental Health Task Force on Staff and Client Safety. Available online at www.mass.gov/eohhs/docs/dmh/report-safety-task-force.doc (accessed October 3, 2013).

Bazelon Center for Mental Health Law (2011) Funding for Mental Health Services and Programs. Available online at www.bazelon.org/LinkClick.aspx?fileticket=GzmAbAweikQ%3Dandtabid=436 (accessed October 3, 2013).

Breggin, P. (1991) *Toxic Psychiatry*. New York: St. Martin's Press.

Cooper, D. (1971) *The Death of the Family*. New York: Pantheon Books.

Corsini, R. (ed.) (1981). *Handbook of Innovative Psychotherapies*. New York: Wiley.

Earley, P. (2006) *Crazy*. New York: G. P. Putnam's Sons.

Foucault, M. (1988) *Madness and Civilization: A History of Insanity in the Age of Reason*. Trans. R. Howard. New York: Vintage Books.

Freire, P. (1970) *Pedagogy of the Oppressed*. New York: Continuum.

French, L. (1987) Victimization of the mentally ill: An unintended consequence of deinstitutionalization. *Social Work*, 32 (6): 502–5.

Ginsberg, T. (2006) Donations tie drug firms and nonprofits. *Philadelphia Inquirer*, May 28. Available online at http://mindfreedom.org/campaign/media/mf/inquirer-on-drug-firms/ (accessed October 3, 2013).

Goffman, E. (1970) *Asylums: Essays on the Social Situation of Mental Patients And Other Inmates*. Chicago, IL: Aldine.

Kim, M. M., Ford, J. D., Howard, D. L., and Bradford, D. W. (2010) Assessing trauma, substance abuse, and mental health in a sample of homeless men. *Health and Social Work*, 35 (1): 39–48.

Laing, R. D. (1965) *The Divided Self: An Existential Study in Sanity and Madness*. Harmondsworth: Penguin Books.

Lamb, H. (2001) Deinstitutionalization at the beginning of the new millennium. *New Directions For Mental Health Services*, 90: 3–20.

Martín-Baró, I., Aron, A., and Corne, S. (1994) *Writings for a Liberation Psychology*. Cambridge, MA: Harvard University Press.

NCH (2006) *Mental Illness and Homelessness*. NCH Fact Sheet No. 5. Washington DC: National Coalition for the Homeless. Available online at www.nationalhomeless.org/publications/facts/Mental_Illness.pdf (accessed October 14, 2013).

Perron, B., Alexander-Eitzman, B., Gillespie, D. F., and Pollio, D. (2008) Modeling the mental health effects of victimization among homeless persons. *Social Science and Medicine*, 67 (9): 1475–9.

SAMHSA (2012) National report finds one-in-five Americans experienced mental illness in the past year [press release]. Available online at www.samhsa.gov/newsroom/advisories/1201185326.aspx (accessed October 3, 2013).

Stefan, S. (2001) *Unequal Rights: Discrimination Against People with Mental Disabilities and The Americans with Disabilities Act*. Washington, DC: American Psychological Association.

Sullivan, W. (1992) Reclaiming the community: The strengths perspective and deinstitutionalization. *Social Work*, 37 (3): 204–9.

Sun, A. (2012) Helping homeless individuals with co-occurring disorders: The four components. *Social Work*, 57 (1): 23–37.

Szasz, T. (1977) *Psychiatric Slavery*. New York: Free Press.

5

LIBERATION HEALTH AND WOMEN SURVIVORS OF VIOLENCE

Ann Fleck-Henderson and Jacqueline Savage Borne

Introduction and institutional context of the case to be presented

The work described here occurs in a dedicated domestic violence program in a large urban teaching hospital. Safe Horizons (not its real name) is a hospital-based domestic violence intervention service that provides advocacy[1] and counseling to patients, employees, family or anyone eligible to use the hospital who is experiencing intimate partner abuse. The social workers who staff the program are referred to as advocates. The program is also a training site for Master of Social Work interns. One of the authors, JSB, is an advocate in the program and the clinician in this case. The other author is her "mentor" in liberation health and a retired social work professor. Both were attracted to liberation health practice because of its fit with the assumptions and values of the battered women's movement.

Intimate violence in the United States

The most recent and best US data on the prevalence of intimate violence against men and women comes from the Centers for Disease Control and Prevention's National Intimate and Sexual Violence Survey (CDC 2011). These data indicate that about one third of women and one-quarter of men in the United States have experienced rape, physical violence and/or stalking by an intimate partner in their lifetime. About one-quarter of women and one in seven men have experienced severe physical violence, e.g. hit with a fist or large object, beaten, slammed against something. Women are more likely to have experienced multiple forms of violence. Important for public health is the finding that 81 percent of women who experienced intimate violence of any sort reported significant long- or short-term impacts related to the violence, while about 35 percent of men reported such effects. The woman whose story is presented in this chapter is a survivor of multiple forms of violence who is dealing with the effects of that experience in the context of her other life circumstances and social positions.

Literature review

Three interrelated strands of literature inform a liberation model of work with women: Feminist psychology, liberation psychology, and, particularly for work with women in abusive relationships, the literature on domestic violence or intimate partner violence. All three of these bodies of thought, and their related approaches to social, community and personal change, have developed primarily since the 1960s. This section describes critical ideas from a few seminal works in each of the three traditions. Common themes and points of difference follow.

From radical feminist psychology

Feminism has a long history, in which the period of the 1960s and 1970s is usually referred to as the "second wave." Within this period, radical feminism is often distinguished from "reformist feminism" (hooks 2000) or "liberal feminism" (Kemp and Brandwein 2010). The latter came to focus on equality of opportunity within the existing systems, while the former focused on changing the culture. Liberation health is more closely connected in its focus and goals to radical feminism.

Although she did not call herself that, Jean Baker Miller was an early radical feminist. Her 1976 book, *Toward a New Psychology of Women*, begins with a chapter entitled, "Domination-subordination." Subordinates and dominants are people or groups of people who are permanently unequal, as opposed to children/parents or students/teachers who are intended to be temporarily unequal. Dominants become the model for "normal," see subordinates as inferior, and "usually define one or more acceptable roles" for subordinates (Miller 1976: 6). A central idea is that these positions of dominance and subordination create psychological charac-teristics, both strengths and deficits, in both groups. Subordinates, in this case women, whose survival often depends on pleasing dominants, orient to dominants' (in this case men's) needs and have a much better knowledge of men than men do of women. Women, and subordinates in general, are more able to tolerate weakness, vulnerability and helplessness than men, or dominants and are more practiced in emotional expression, supporting others' development and cooperation. At the same time, and because of their position as subordinates, they find it difficult to claim their own needs, express anger or engage openly in conflict, as conflict with someone in a dominant position is inherently dangerous (chapter 4). Miller outlines the importance of "reclaiming conflict" in order to confront injustice and promote social change. She also notes that social change is already in process when women dare to examine their own needs and begin to speak out (p. 135): the beginnings of social change are a prerequisite for the personal changes necessary to support further social change. In other words, personal and social changes are intrinsically linked.

Early feminist therapy was based in the idea, shared with all liberation psychologies, that individual psychological pain reflects the powerlessness or oppression of a whole class of people (Morrow and Hawxhurst 1998). Raising ones consciousness means coming to see the social and historical conditions that shape one's personal situation. This critical consciousness is necessary to transform self-blame and self-doubt which the subordinate condition breeds. Consciousness-raising was a central concept for the women's movement of the 1970s. Hence, the well-known feminist slogan: "The personal is political."

Qualitative research on women's development has often used the metaphor of silence and voice to describe women's development of agency (Belenky, Clinchy, Goldberger and Tarule 1997; Belenky, Bond and Weinstock 1991; Goodman, *et al.* 2004: 802). In one study, the most economically, socially and educationally deprived women were least able to know or express views separate from those dictated by often abusive authorities in their lives (Belenky, *et al.* 1986, chapter 1). Building on this observation of silenced women, Belenky, *et al.* (1991) describe a number of projects "dedicated to bringing an excluded group into voice" (p. 4). Some of these projects focused on individual development, some on leadership development, some on community development. First, oppressed women begin to trust their own perspectives and speak out, always in the context of developmental and non-authoritarian relationships; then, in solidarity with others in similar situations they act to change unjust conditions.

bell hooks, influenced by Paulo Freire, writes from a North American and African-American perspective about liberating educational approaches. Particularly valuable to this project is her clarity about racial and class tensions, her ability to maintain feminist solidarity without denying or suppressing critical differences among women. In a chapter titled "Holding my sister's hand: Feminist solidarity" (hooks 1994, chapter 7) she outlines the history of hostility, mistrust and competition between black and white women in this country. Sexual competition and a history of subordinate/dominant relationships (slave/mistress or servant/mistress) are a legacy "shared from generation to generation keeping alive the sense of distance and separation, feelings of suspicion and mistrust" (1994: 101). She states further that "until we can acknowledge the negative history which shapes and informs our contemporary interaction, there can be no honest, meaningful dialogue" (ibid, p.102). We are choosing bell hooks to represent many writers who have worked to correct early feminism's relative blindness to the power of class, race and other differences among women.

From liberation psychology

Liberation psychology assumes that the psychological suffering of anyone in an oppressed position is in some part a function of that oppression. The cycle of liberation includes personal, interpersonal or collective, and political change (e.g. Moane 2003: 97, 2011: 89). There cannot be real health without change in the oppressive conditions. This is not a linear process (psychological to collective to political), but truly a circular one. Freire emphasizes the necessity of action to change concrete oppressive conditions as essential for psychological liberation. However, some psychological liberation, through analysis of the conditions of oppression, may be needed first (Freire 2005: 48, 61–4, e.g.), as the conditions of oppression create psychological patterns, such as a sense of inferiority, or self-doubt, which reduce the capacity to act (Moane, 2003, p.96–7; 2011, p. 88). Although personal transformation is an essential component of liberation, the focus is always on the collective. Each level of change requires connection with other people who are similarly situated. Only together, in dialogue, can people analyze, act and reflect. Although the analysis and resistance must originate with those who are oppressed, it may need to be catalyzed by someone who is outside the oppressed group. (See e.g., Freire, "Pedagogy of the Heart," Chapter 8 in Freire, A. and Macedo 1998: 273, last para.).

Critical consciousness, i.e., being able to see (or read) the social, political and historical conditions that shape one's experience, is essential to liberation. It is through an analysis of these conditions that people in oppressed groups can realize the structural sources of much of their difficulty and subsequently find ways to act to change these conditions. Critical consciousness of one's own social structural position is also necessary for anyone working with oppressed people. Particularly important for those who would be allies is consciousness of the limited nature of one's own perspective as a (usually more privileged) outsider. Those who are in subordinate positions are the only ones who can truly see what needs to be changed and what they can realistically do about it.

From the anti-domestic violence literature

The case we discuss in this chapter is that of a woman dealing with domestic violence whom the social worker meets in the context of a dedicated domestic violence service. The roots of today's services for victims of intimate violence are in a liberation movement. To quote one of that movement's pioneers: "Without an ideology and a practice based in the hope of liberation for all women, including those who face the greatest discrimination and have the fewest resources, a movement will flounder and move in more conservative directions" (Schechter 1982: 6).

Today, services for those affected by intimate violence (victims and perpetrators) come in many forms, more and less consistent with the movement's earlier goals and practices, reflecting a tension between movement organizations and service organizations, self-help and professional approaches (Davies, Lyon and Monti-Catania 1998; Goodman and Epstein 2009; Shepard and Pence 1999: 7; Schechter 1982: 110–11). The movement's success in garnering attention and resources came at a considerable price. As domestic violence services have received government and other funding outside the movement, they have become increasingly professionalized, fragmented and narrow. What began as a liberation movement has, to a large degree, become part of health and criminal justice bureaucracies.

Goodman and Epstein (2009) give an excellent short history of these develop-ments. While respectfully acknowledging the value of current services, they indicate their implicit limits and unintended negative consequences for many women, as well as the barriers to real social change. "As professional services became the chief offering of domestic violence organizations, political activism moved toward the periphery" (Goodman and Epstein 2009: 41). In conclusion, they propose three basic principles: listening to individual women's voices, promo-ting supportive communities, and facilitating economic empowerment (Goodman and Epstein 2009: 6, 135). Economic empowerment includes challenging structural barriers to empowerment; e.g. privatized nuclear families, acceptance of violence, and lack of available day care, flexible work, health care.

The principles specified by Goodman and Epstein (2009) are consistent with the early battered women's movement, radical feminism and liberation psychology. Although they may be difficult to enact in agencies as currently structured and funded, it is possible to take a liberation or social justice perspective within a traditional agency (Almeida, Dolan-Del Vecchio, and Parker 2007b, p. 176). Advo-cates and social workers in traditional organizations are often creative in maintaining a survivor-centered stance, supporting survivor groups, and building community connections that can be sustained beyond the advocate's role with the woman.

A few programs working with families dealing with violence are structured specifically to embody social justice principles. One is the clinic of the Just Therapy team in New Zealand (Waldegrave, Tamasese, Tuhaka, and Campbell 2003). Another is the Institute for Family Services in New Jersey, which is the home of the cultural context model (Almeida and Lockhard 2005; Almeida, et al. 2007a and 2007b).

The New Zealand team works with people of Maori, Pacific Island and Euro-pean heritage. Structurally, the agency is organized in cultural "sections," each of which also has men's and women's groups. Work with Maori or Pacific Island people is accountable to the relevant cultural section. Work that involves women is accountable to women on the staff. The social, cultural, historical and political context of a family is intrinsic to the work.

The guiding principles of the cultural context model are critical consciousness, accountability, and empowerment:

> The model offers solutions to families by connecting them to a community that promotes liberation. As clients gain knowledge and support from the community, they work within this collective to challenge the systems of power, privilege, and oppression that are the foundation of many presenting problems.
>
> (Almeida, et al. 2007b: 179)

From a liberation perspective, survivor groups are a critical context for dialogue, reflection and collective action. Those experiencing domestic abuse are often iso-lated from relationships outside the family, so groups become especially important for healing.

Summary

The three traditions sampled above share the assumption that personal troubles reflect political issues. Individual suffering is shaped by social and political conditions; in particular, the condition of oppression in a hierarchical social structure, and, as with critical theories generally, social structures are seen as inevitably hierarchical. Each of these traditions sees individual change as essential, but not sufficient, for social change. In different language each emphasizes three levels of change: personal, interpersonal and social/cultural.

Each of the traditions depends on social analysis, what the early women's movement called "consciousness-raising" and liberation psychology calls "conscientization" (Freire 2005: 35, note 1; Montero and Sonn 2009: 56). Social analysis allows people to make the social conditions of their oppression conscious objects of their awareness and attention (Friere 2005: 109) and, thereby, to see themselves as part of a larger collective of people who share an unjust situation.

A second component of the three traditions is reflection with others who share the same situation. A collective or group process, in which people *themselves* name their experience and identify unifying themes in their situations is an essential element. Individual work with a professional cannot have the same power as reflection and dialogue with similarly situated others. If for no other reason, a professional therapeutic relationship is, itself, a hierarchical relationship in which the client is often in the subordinate position. More importantly from a liberation psychology perspective, the collective has to be at the center of change.

Each of the traditions also calls to change the culture through social action. The action element is central to liberation psychology. What particular form it would take depends on the collective analysis of conditions and decisions to act. Radical feminist psychology, including the literature of the early battered women's movement, speaks to the need for change in both cultural attitudes and social policies, but seems less clear than liberation psychology in its directive to social action. The two programs mentioned, which are among the more radical of domestic violence intervention programs, focus action largely on holding the more powerful (dominant) group accountable to their peers and to the less dominant through specific interventions in families and communities. As most domestic violence programs in the US, including the one discussed in this chapter, work only with survivors or only with abusers, that form of social action is not available to them.

Case presentation

Introduction to the context

Safe Horizons, the institutional context for this work, is voluntary, confidential, free of charge, and does not utilize insurance. Services are offered from an empowerment-based feminist approach, and advocates (social workers) tailor assistance to the client's desire to engage. Services range from crisis intervention to long-term advocacy, counseling and group work. The program does not diagnose its clients and does not chart any notes in the hospital's medical record system.

Referral and presenting issue

Alyce (a fictional name) is a 59-year-old woman of Jamaican descent and birth. She came to the United States when she was 12 and speaks with a strong Jamaican accent. Alyce identifies as Protestant, specifically Seventh Day Adventist. She married a southern Baptist African-American man at age 18 and had three children who are now adults, two daughters and a son.

Alyce was referred by her primary-care physician from one of the hospital's clinics. Her doctor reported she suffered from recurrent headaches as well as chronic back pain and body aches. She also had contracted genital warts about five years earlier, and, as a result, had often endured periods of visible sores on her forearms and hands. After repeated screenings for domestic abuse by her physician at annual visits, Alyce mentioned that the headaches she gets might be related to times her husband had hit her over many years in their marriage. At that time she agreed to speak with a medical social worker, who then connected her with the Safe Horizons program.

When Alyce initially presented to the program she appeared sad and fearful, using words like "stuck, scared, hopeless and weak." She stated that she was "wasting [advocate's] time," and continually inquired whether there were other women who were more deserving of the program's help. Simultaneously, she expressed doubt that other people had gone through similar issues and made several disparaging comments about herself, blaming herself for "getting into this marriage, and staying in it for so long." Although she spoke quietly and rarely made eye contact, she came in regularly, continued to make follow-up appointments and was engaged in conversation.

Alyce had been married for 41 years and had talked to very few people about the abuse, and to no one about the full history. Over several months, the story emerged of years of physical assaults, including strangulations; also psychological, financial and spiritual abuse.

Current situation

At the time represented in this writing, Alyce had been in the program for over three years. After the first eight months of work with an advocate, Alyce joined a writing group composed of women participating in the program. Alyce has a low literacy level, which initially made her very reluctant to join the group. Once a member, however, she became an active participant and ultimately a leader in this group. Several months after joining, Alyce took out a restraining order to have her husband vacate their home and subsequently worked with an attorney to obtain a separation and eventual divorce. Months later, she participated in a regional conference along with her advocate that highlighted creative approaches to healing from domestic violence. Currently, she is supported on Social Security Disability Insurance, social security, minimal alimony, and financial help from one of her adult children. She continues to see her advocate as needed. The original writing group has ended, and Alyce is thinking about joining another group.

Relevant history

Alyce went to grammar school in Jamaica and had great difficulty in school after she moved to the United States with her mother and grandmother at age 12. She remembered being teased and being very self-conscious about her accent. She attended school until the age of 16, at which time she met her husband, who was 22. He encouraged her to drop out and "prepare for them to marry," which she did. At age 18, she married and gained permanent citizenship through the union. Alyce's three children were born over the next nine years. Alyce has not ever worked steadily. Once her children were all in school, she took on sporadic childcare and cleaning jobs, but reported feeling incompetent and nervous about her performance while she was working. Her husband has worked at the same factory since they met.

About ten years into their marriage, Alyce started attending a Seventh Day Adventist church, which she associated with very positive memories from her upbringing in Jamaica. Her husband disliked the church and accused her of having affairs with men in the church community. Over time, Alyce believed choosing to feel spiritually and emotionally "whole" meant facing the escalation of abuse at home.

Later when Alyce began to contemplate separation and eventually divorce, she described the few close friends she had made at church as being supportive. However, her two older children opposed the separation, saying that their father could not manage without her and that it was difficult to think of their parents not together after all this time. Alyce describes continually feeling guilty and confused as a result.

Once Alyce began talking openly about the abuse she disclosed details of forced sex, although she did not term it as such. There were repeated assaults when her husband specifically aimed to hit her in the head and face. Alyce recounted an incident when her husband came home from work and told her that his boss, a white man, had used a racial slur when reprimanding him at the factory. Her response struck him as being unsympathetic and "disloyal to your own people." He then physically beat her to the point she was almost unconscious.

Sometimes Alyce screamed during assaults and felt quite sure neighbors in their housing complex could hear her, but no one ever called the police or approached her to ask if she was okay. Alyce dialed 911 during a few particularly frightening incidents, but she always recanted out of fear when the police arrived. She recalls the responding officers telling her husband to calm down and inviting him to take a walk around the block.

With support from the writing group, Alyce obtained a restraining order, and her husband moved out of their home. He did, however, continue to come to the house and call her which involved more subtle forms of emotional abuse. Alyce frequently said there were many ways the physical abuse felt "less crazy-making."

"When he hit me, it would leave a mark I could show people. When he played with my mind, and I tried to explain it to someone, I felt like I sounded crazy." She eventually worked with a legal aid attorney to obtain a divorce and also decided to sell her house.

Alyce continues to see her advocate as needed. She often will go periods of time without connecting and then calls or responds to outreach, finding it helpful to discuss current feelings or fears. She reports that she is freer, less in fear and less isolated, although she has future goals of connecting with more friends and resources in her community.

Formulation

Alyce, a 59-year-old US citizen born in Jamaica, sought services because of a history of domestic abuse from her husband of 41 years. She reported being stuck in an abusive marriage, afraid to make a change, ashamed of herself because of the abuse and feeling like a failure generally, someone who "got no respect." Alyce also suffers from chronic pain, headaches and a sexually transmitted infection.

Alyce has a history of physical, sexual, spiritual, psychological, and financial abuse from her husband. Her sense of shame and guilt reflects her husband's constant messages, as well as the culture's construction of abuse as a personal and private issue rather than a product of social and cultural forces. This construction of domestic abuse as a private matter is seen also in responses to her cries for help, both from the police and from her neighbors. Traditional gender roles and dominant cultural messaging shape Alyce's perspective: assuming that women are responsible for relationships; taking the blame for marital difficulties; leaving high school to prioritize "preparing to marry"; and assuming her husband's entitlement to her personal and sexual services. Such gender roles also shape her children's perception that he cannot take care of himself without her and their resulting opposition to her separating from the marriage.

Personal factors which shape her presenting concerns include her low level of education and literacy, her accented speech, minimal employment through her life and small number of important personal relationships. Each of these is linked to institutional and cultural factors. Starting school in the United States when she was 12, Alyce's initial trouble with the language contributed to her school failures. Her accent has also made it more difficult to negotiate the court system. In a culture that values literacy very highly, her low literacy is a handicap and stigmatizing. Similarly, her lack of employable skills and minimal employment history are particularly demeaning in a culture that values paid productivity and does not include home making and child rearing as such. Her relative isolation, except for some relationships at church, is a product of her husband's efforts, her lack of work-based relationships and the cultural value on individualism and self-sufficiency which may inhibit neighborhood connections. Finally, the cultural definition of family as a bounded nuclear unit, rather than an extended family, has contributed to Alyce's isolation.

We should note in our formulation that those working with Alyce in our program are white and US born. Consistent with our institutional and cultural values on privacy and confidentiality, we have no contact with her family, church or neighborhood.

Interventions

We have organized the intervention section first by the goal or hope for the intervention, and within each of these by chronology. The first person voice is that of the social worker/advocate. In the early months of her work in the program, Alyce saw her advocate individually. Later, she joined a writing group of other survivors, while continuing individual work.

Consciousness-raising: Broadening analysis of the issue beyond the personal and individual

Our beginning work included education (introducing new information and deconstructing some dominant cultural messages), support and relationship building. I introduced the power and control wheel[2] early on, as a tool to help explain the dynamics of domestic abuse, to validate my assertion that a significant number of people endure this in their relationship, and to begin to expand Alyce's understanding of her situation beyond the individual/personal level. Once we had spent some time discussing the wheel, I asked Alyce to think with me about creating her own wheel, to produce a visual representation of the abuse in her relationship. My goal, once she began to have a context for the global/systemic nature of this issue, was to help her

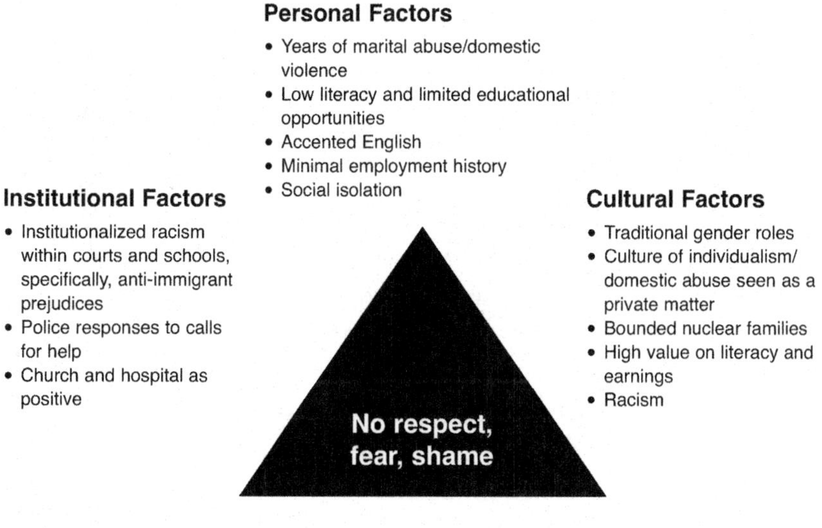

Personal Factors

- Years of marital abuse/domestic violence
- Low literacy and limited educational opportunities
- Accented English
- Minimal employment history
- Social isolation

Institutional Factors

- Institutionalized racism within courts and schools, specifically, anti-immigrant prejudices
- Police responses to calls for help
- Church and hospital as positive

Cultural Factors

- Traditional gender roles
- Culture of individualism/ domestic abuse seen as a private matter
- Bounded nuclear families
- High value on literacy and earnings
- Racism

No respect, fear, shame

FIGURE 5.1 Liberation health and women survivors of violence
Source: Jacqueline Savage Borne and Ann Fleck-Henderson

begin to think beyond the definitions others used to characterize abuse and to feel the right to define her own experiences. Rather than the words "power and control" at the center of the wheel, Alyce chose the phrases "no respect" and "fear and shame," and was able to list details of several subheadings that helped to describe her experiences of abuse over the years (see Figure 5.2).

Central to this beginning work was introducing the idea of internalized abuse. Alyce came to our work making many self-deprecating comments about herself and her own worth, often not even realizing she was doing so. Examples included comments such as, "He gets frustrated with me because I don't know how to do so many things around the house. I blame myself for never learning." "My kids tell me to speak up for myself and I should – I set such a terrible example for them." In response to my comments, she acknowledged that these were judgments that her husband had repeatedly made over the course of her entire adult life. I suggested that it would make sense that she would not only believe him, but eventually internalize those judgments as her own.

Later, in the writing group, Alyce got support to expand her analysis to issues of race and class. For instance, when Alyce recounted her experience in court to get a restraining order, she characterized it as stressful and frightening to tell such

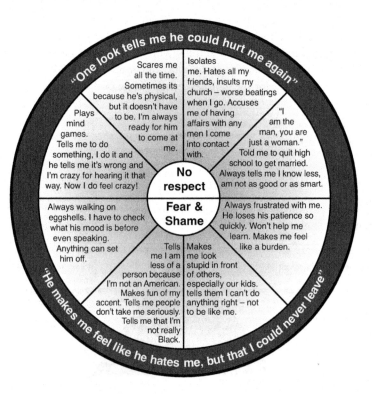

FIGURE 5.2 A's personal power and control wheel

Source: Jacqueline Savage Borne and Ann Fleck-Henderson

intimate details in front of an open court room of strangers, and that the judge felt intimidating. Alyce had been questioned by the judge, and twice the judge asked her to "speak up," noting that because of "her very strong accent" it was difficult to understand her. The conversation was initially about the power the judge held to give or not give a restraining order. The discussion then went more deeply into the actual comment he had made about Alyce's accent. Questions were raised in the group whether he would have done this if she were a white woman, or a white man, or someone who appeared to be more privileged. Parallel questions were posed as to whether he would have made that comment as a man of color, a white woman, or a woman of color. Other group members pointed out that his remark about her accent was in fact racist and an abuse of his power. Alyce had initially accepted the dominant cultural message that an accent is a personal deficit. Her understanding of this incident evolved as the group deconstructed that message, and she talked earnestly about feeling empowered to label the incident as oppressive. This was a clear example of the collective power of fellow survivors. I had posed some of these questions to Alyce in our individual counseling sessions, and though there was some discussion, the group conversation led to a deeper level of awareness, support and eventual action. As a white woman in a helping professional role who does not identify as an abuse survivor, I could not engage Alyce in the same way as her fellow survivors of abuse.

Still later, when Alyce considered separating from her husband, the group discussed the difficulty of being single, especially after many years of marriage. The group facilitators asked members to think about what messages they had been given by their own families, cultural groups and larger society about being unmarried, or becoming divorced, i.e. to identify the dominant "world views." This discussion again broadened Alyce's analysis to look at internalized messages not only from her husband, but also from the larger culture.

As part of my ongoing work with Alyce, I have done my best to attend to the power dynamics within our own relationship. As part of our initial engagement, I raised the issue of the differences in our cultural/racial identity and asked her directly how this is for her, as she had already referred to negative experiences with white people. When we were looking together at the power and control wheel, I noted that power can exist not only in abusive relationships, but in helping ones as well. I hoped to direct her thinking beyond individual traits to the power of structured hierarchies and also to acknowledge that there may well be times that I would inadvertently misuse the power I held in our relationship. Although she did not want to discuss this initially, we have been able to have some conversation about it as issues between us have arisen. For instance, Alyce often has not called me when she wants to cancel or reschedule an appointment, because she feels "bad." Originally, I repetitively told her she should not feel that way, as it was her choice when and how to work with our program. That reassurance changed nothing, and I realized that the power I inherently hold in the relationship could be contributing to her fear of disappointing me, not living up to my expectations or "rules." Although we both acknowledge this, it does not make the dynamic disappear.

Developing a sense of solidarity, connection and inclusion

The early individual work helped Alyce to begin to see herself as a member of a class of people, both women and survivors of abuse. This shift in her thinking was not yet actualized in her relationships, which would be an important next step. The program had a writing-focused support group, created after requests from past groups for more creatively oriented ways to heal from abuse and connect with other survivors. In this group members were invited to write during (and beyond) group sessions, driven by a curriculum of exercises. Participants had the choice to share their pieces, which fueled discussion and hopefully created a mutual aid process.

When I suggested to Alyce that she try out this group, she was very tentative about participating. She cited her low literacy level as the primary reason, as well as her general reluctance to tell her story in what she perceived as a public setting. I let her know it was completely her choice, and I would respect a decision not to attend, recognizing the risks involved. After about a month of weighing the pros and cons of attending, Alyce decided to attend a session, assured she did not need to participate any more than she chose and also did not need to return.

Alyce was quiet and mostly observant in the first group session, and later said one of the reasons she felt comfortable there is that no one judged her for doing so. She began to take small risks, like talking longer during a check-in, or briefly offering her thoughts when another participant shared a story. Alyce and I had weekly debriefs in our individual sessions about her feelings regarding the group. What she recounted as most important was the conversations she had with participants in the group. As an example, Alyce decided to abstain from writing exercises the first few months of group. When another member asked her if she was going to try writing, she became reserved and appeared embarrassed. The participant continued to gently push, saying "I bet you're a great writer, you have such a pretty way of talking." Alyce then shared that she didn't have a lot of confidence in her writing skill. She and I had talked privately about her dictating writing to me, whether in group or individually. She shared this idea with the group in that session, and they reacted very positively. Using the exercise we were doing that day, "Write about the differences between being lonely and being alone," she began experimenting with dictating different words and phrases. She recounted finding the process as well as the positive reinforcement she received from other members invigorating and empowering.

Alyce continued to attend this group for several months during a crucial decision-making point in her relationship. After several conversations and nonjudgmental support from the other women in the group, she decided to seek a restraining order against her husband, forcing him to vacate their home. She talked through each aspect of the decision with members and reported back after she successfully obtained the order.

The decision about seeking a restraining order was an exceedingly difficult one with which Alyce struggled, going back and forth several times. There was no certainty about how her husband would react; whether an order would be a deterrent to his battering or would cause escalation of that abuse. Weekly individual work continued as well as the group discussions. I encouraged Alyce to bring the questions she was posing in our conversations to her fellow group members, and she gained increasing comfort in doing so. When she and I created a list of pros and cons on seeking an order, the potency of that process seemed far greater when she could debrief it with other group participants who had had similar experiences. Alyce was able to go ahead with obtaining the order when these discussions yielded the conclusion that the risks of going to court were outweighed by the potential benefits. Recognizing, processing and acknowledging that these risks would not disappear seemed an essential step in her moving forward. The group's ability to stand in solidarity with her through this process enabled her to do it.

A related conversation in the group concerned the messages members had received about being unmarried in our culture. Women in the group were of varying ages and relationship statuses, and the majority of members were women of color. When Alyce was in the process of contemplating the order and thereby forcing her husband to leave their home, a fellow member asked her the simple question "what would it be like for you to sleep alone in your house after all these years?." That one inquiry opened up a series of fruitful conversations about both the grieving involved with ending an abusive relationship, as well as the difficulty of seeing oneself in the world as single, particularly after being married for some time. One woman shared that though she had been divorced for three years, she still had trouble saying it out loud. She said she even would try to practice in places like a grocery store, where no one knew her, saying something to the effect of "I only need a few things because it's just me at home. I'm divorced." Being divorced still felt difficult and subject to societal judgment. Members' postulating about why this was so hard led to their identifying the dominant messaging women receive about the importance of being coupled, and the shame they can feel about voluntarily leaving a relationship. One participant said, "Sometimes I wish my husband had died. Not because he treated me so badly, but because it would be easier to say I was a widow than divorced." Group facilitators asked the women what they thought led to these strong cultural messages and whether the power and control wheel was related. The women then identified different ways in which male economic and social dominance was supported by traditional marriage and also led them to feel more vulnerable and less worthy when single.

Taking action

When Alyce brought her experience with the district court to the group, other participants talked about their court experiences that felt discriminatory and degrading. A group discussion ensued about what action could possibly be taken to address these situations. A collective decision was made to research court watch programs, and the group worked together on strategizing how to report these events.

Another notable incident occurred when Alyce was asked by her attorney to request her medical record for purposes of her divorce proceedings. She talked first with me individually about being surprised to see documentation written by her doctor recounting the details of abuse she had disclosed. Alyce acknowledged that in fact these notes were helpful in her legal proceedings, but that it felt "strange" to see them after all this time. I encouraged her to bring this to the group, which she did. Members were intrigued and began to talk about their realization that they have never seen their own medical records. In conjunction with conversation with the group facilitators, they made plans to request their individual medical records and review them as a group. Facilitators also offered to help make connections with appropriate entities at the hospital for members to offer thoughts about this should they choose to do so. Whereas Alyce's initial feeling had been "doctors just need to do what they need to do," the group process helped her to feel entitled to know what is in her records and be informed before things are written. The group talked about the power differences they constantly feel with doctors, and considered both the difficulty and worth in talking directly with their physicians about their feelings on this and other matters.

The clearest example of collective action was the group's production of a book of writings, intended to help new participants in our program. The facilitators did not begin the group with a product in mind; it was conceived solely as a way to gain healing through creativity. Once the group was underway, participants began talking together about the idea of a book. We encouraged and nurtured the idea, but did not lead it. Through collective discussion, group members decided we should have an end product that included their writings, and that we also should invite program advocates and medical doctors to write about their experiences of helping survivors. Further, as some group members had difficulty writing, either because of their reluctance to do so or due to literacy issues, another idea emerged. Participants suggested adding a photography component. Each member was given a disposable camera to take pictures, with certain safety considerations in place, and these pictures came back to the group to inspire poems, prose or other pieces. An example was a picture taken of a newspaper dispenser that simply read "FREE." This inspired a group discussion about what it meant to be truly free and a piece that Alyce consequently wrote through dictation to an advocate. It read in part: "And just free to be myself and to love myself."

Together with her advocate, Alyce has spoken at a statewide conference that highlighted creative approaches to healing from domestic violence. This required significant conversation about potential risk and safety concerns in telling her story in a more public setting. Eventually she decided that with the proper planning she could feel physically safe from her ex-partner doing so, and she could feel emotionally safe being so public, because the perceived rewards felt worthwhile. Alyce has additionally given permission for her poem to be part of hospital-wide and community presentations that train physicians and other medical providers on the issue of domestic violence. She talks about the importance of her voice being part of a bigger movement, and the ways in which this has helped her own continued healing.

Summary

The work with Alyce involved a shift in her understanding of the abuse she had suffered, through both new information and deconstructing dominant cultural messages; connection with a group of survivors of domestic abuse and their (staff) allies, leading to a sense of solidarity with a group and a movement; and collective actions to change the social conditions which support various forms of oppression, leading to an increased sense of personal power. These actions included the group's writing a small book which might inspire hope in other survivors, Alyce's speaking to a conference of professionals to improve their understanding of the experience of survivors of domestic abuse, and potential social action initiatives in the court system and in the hospital.

Reflections

In this section of the chapter, we reflect on the differences of this work from more typical approaches to work with survivors of violence and the challenges of doing this kind of work. The second part of this section is written in the first person voice of JSB and the first part in a more impersonal voice; both express our discussions with each other and our shared thoughts.

Alyce's understanding shifted from seeing her situation as her individual problem, largely a result of her own failings, to seeing it as a part of a general issue of abuses of power, specifically of men against women, but also of other figures (judge, doctor) with positions of power in social hierarchies. This shift was facilitated first by her advocate's use of the power and control wheel, her sharing of the experiences of other women, her introduction of concepts like male entitlement and internalized abuse. In those ways, seeds were sown by the advocate, but it took the group of other women to consolidate a new perspective and new ability to take action. In our view, the group was necessary for Alyce to fully feel her own power. In addition to its role in Alyce's developing her own "voice," it provided a trustworthy source of relevant wisdom and tips, and it helped her to see the social roots of her abusive relationship in ways that the advocate alone could not.

This was a particularly powerful group in a program that does not have group work as a central or necessary component. Alyce's experience, as well as our understanding of liberation psychology, lead us to wonder to what degree these shifts could have occurred without the group. Although support groups are core parts of many domestic violence programs, advocacy at many hospital or court-based programs is, at this point, conceived primarily as a one-to one relationship, and linking to groups is not an intrinsic part of the work. That may be changing in this agency as the staff becomes increasingly impressed with the importance of groups.

The individual client–advocate relationship is often one that crosses education and class differences and sometimes also racial/ethnic differences. The advocate in our case addressed with Alyce the race, class and educational differences between them. She could not, however, neutralize the power disparities. That power difference in a relationship intended to be empowering seems an inevitable tension.

The agency does not normally include the family or other community in the work, thus enacting and reflecting the individualistic assumptions of much of social work. A central aim of the program is to help a client decrease the isolation that inevitably comes with domestic violence, and conversely expand their network of social support and create a sense of solidarity within a larger community. This goal is subverted if the client becomes singularly "dependent" on the advocate or program. Ideally, liberation health would support the woman in building and/or developing relationships beyond the agency. In this case, those relationships, at least so far, are all within the context of the agency.

Liberation health work does not fit easily with third-party payments and is usually dependent on grants and other funders. This agency has the advantage of being funded as part of a hospital's community service mission. That structure allows the advocates considerable freedom in duration of contact with clients and in the nature of the work they do. Given the service-driven and fragmented nature of most services for survivors of intimate abuse, this freedom to follow the lead of the survivor makes liberation work at least possible. It is, however, vulnerable to a change in priorities of its host institution, a major teaching hospital.

We end this section with some thoughts in the first person voice of JSB.

Thoughts

I have noticed throughout my years of domestic violence work that clients often ask us as advocates why abusers abuse. Typically, our "answers" go back to the concepts of power and control, and in the case of heterosexual couples, male entitlement and patriarchal societal messaging. These are essential messages, and, as we can see in Alyce's story, not intuitively obvious to most survivors. However, I have often felt that clients were looking for more when they asked this. Often, it is clear in the survivor's story that the abusive person is also suffering from poverty and/or racism, and, if he is male, he may himself be acting partly on cultural messages of what it means to be a strong man. How do such perceptions fit into our work with those who are victims of abuse?

With Alyce, these questions came to mind particularly around the story of her husband's assaulting her after he had been racially discriminated against at his workplace. Alyce was notably struck by his claim that she was betraying "her people" by "not taking his side," and wanted to discuss this. I acknowledged that he was a victim of racism, which was wrong, and gave a clear message this did not excuse his assault. However, I focused on her safety, the health effects of enduring such significant physical violence, and essentially gave the message that this was yet another example of her husband's attributing his abuse to someone else.

In reflecting on my work with Alyce and becoming immersed in the liberation model, I have new questions about that response and others like it. On the one hand, it is critical for victims to see that the abuser is responsible for the abuse and should be held accountable. This is a central idea in domestic violence advocacy. Like Alyce, most survivors blame themselves and/or forces beyond the abuser's control (his parents, his drinking, mental health, etc.) We are reluctant to provide excuses for the abuser or contribute to the survivor's feelings of responsibility for the abuse or the abuser. Accordingly, with Alyce I always attempted to point to her husband's responsibility for the abuse, and her lack of culpability in it, and this did feel truly helpful to her.

On the other hand, I recognize now that this is a somewhat singular perspective that does not leave room to discuss "reasons" for her husband's behavior. In some ways, it parallels the early women's movement's singular focus on gender and neglect of race and class. Would it have been helpful to explore the powerlessness and impotency her husband was feeling in that moment and his need to align with another person of color? In our work, we talked a good deal about Alyce's feelings of oppression around cultural identity, racism and oppression, but I was admittedly mostly race-silent on anything having to do with her husband. I am considering now how a conversation about an abuser's potential oppression could fit into this discussion. The concern for weakening the message of personal accountability is clear and legitimate, but the benefits of exploring these issues also seem apparent to me as I reflect on this work.

In conclusion

Current advocacy practice with survivors of violence is consistent with liberation health principles in some respects, but not in all. Both practices frame intimate violence as a cultural and political issue, not simply a personal one. Both counter the internalized abuse of victims. As practiced at Safe Horizons, advocacy is survivor-centered in a way that is not supported in many other settings. Even in this setting, current practice lacks the consistent emphasis of liberation health on collective experience and on social action. Our cultural bias toward individualism is reflected in the priority given to one-on-one work over group work and work in the community. Group work is often seen as healing and providing support and mutual aid; too rarely is it used as a forum for analysis and challenge of oppressive conditions and practices. Finally, we raise the question how survivor-focused work might include analysis of the social forces and cultural messages which also shape the abuser's experience.

Notes

1   Advocacy is an empowerment-based, client-centered approach that blends non-judgmental support with directive feedback and validation. Domestic violence advocacy views risk assessment, safety planning and comprehensive connections to resources and options as core elements. Advocacy is rooted in the client/survivor as expert on his/her own situation and the expectation that the helping professional will build upon and honor that expertise.

2   The power and control wheel is widely used in domestic violence services. See www.ncdsv.org/images/PowerControlwheelNOSHADING.pdf for the standard power and control wheel.

References

Almeida, R. V., Dolan-Del Vecchio, K., and Parker, L. (2007a) *Transformative Family Therapy: Just Families in a Just Society*. Boston, MA: Pearson Education.

Almeida, R. V., Dolan-Del Vecchio, K., and Parker, L. (2007b) Foundation concepts for social justice-based therapy: critical consciousness, accountability, and empowerment. Chapter 8 in Aldarondo, E. (ed.) *Advancing Social Justice Through Clinical Practice*. Mahwah, NJ: Lawrence Erlbaum.

Almeida, R., and Lockard, J. (2005) The cultural context model: A new paradigm for accountability, empowerment, and the development of critical consciousness Against domestic violence. In N. Sokoloff (ed.), *Domestic Violence at the Margins: Readings on Race, Class, Gender, and Culture*. New Brunswick, NJ: Rutgers University Press, pp. 301–20.

Belenky, M. F., Bond, L., and Weinstock, J. (1991) A tradition that has no name: Nurturing the development of people, families, and communities. New York, NY: Basic Books.

Belenky, M. F., Clinchy, B., Goldberger, N., and Tarule, J. (1997) *Women's Ways of Knowing: The Development of Self, Voice, and Mind*. (10th anniv. edn.) New York: Basic Books.

CDC (2011) *The National Intimate Partner and Sexual Violence Survey: 2010 Summary Report*. Atlanta, GA: Centers for Disease Control and Prevention. Available online at www.cdc.gov/violenceprevention/nisvs/ (accessed October 3, 2013).

Davies, J., Lyon, E., and Monti-Catania, D. (1998) *Safety Planning With Battered Women: Complex Lives/Difficult Choices*. Sage Series on Violence against Women. Thousand Oaks, CA: Sage.

Freire, P. (2005) *Pedagogy of the Oppressed*. (30th anniv. edn.) Trans. Myra Bergman Ramos. New York: Continuum.

Freire, A. and Macedo, D. (1998) *The Paulo Freire Reader*. New York: Continuum International.

Goodman, L. and Epstein, D. (2009) *Listening to Battered Women: A Survivor-Centered Approach to Advocacy, Mental Health and Justice*. Washington, DC: American Psychological Association.

Goodman, L., Liang, B., Helms, J., Latta, R., Sparks, E., and Weintraub, S. (2004) Training counseling psychologists as social justice agents: Feminist and multicultural principles in action. *The Counseling Psychologist*, 32 (6): 793–837

hooks, b. (2000) *Feminism is for Everybody*. Cambridge, MA: South End Press.

hooks, b. (1994) *Teaching to Transgress*. New York, NY: Routledge.

Kemp, S. P. and Brandwein, R. (2010) Feminisms and social work in the United States: An intertwined history. *Affilia* 25: 341–64.

Moane, G. (1999, 2011) *Gender and Colonialism: A Psychological Analysis of Oppression and Liberation*. New York, NY: Palgrave Macmillan.

Moane, G. (2003) Bridging the personal and the political: Practices for a liberation psychology. *American Journal of Community Psychology*, 31 (1/2): 91–101.

Miller, J. B. (1976, 1986) *Toward a New Psychology of Women*. Boston, MA: Beacon Press.

Montero, M. and Sonn, C. (eds) (2009) *The Psychology of Liberation: Theory and Applications*. New York: Springer.

Morrow, S. L., and Hawxhurst, D. M. (1998) Feminist therapy: Integrating political analysis in counseling and psychotherapy. *Women and Therapy*, 21 (2): 37–50.

Schechter, S. (1982) *Women and Male Violence: The Visions and Struggles of the Battered Women's Movement*. Boston, MA: South End Press.

Shepard, M. and Pence, E. L. (eds) (1999) *Coordinating Community Responses to Domestic Violence*. Thousand Oaks, CA: Sage Publications, Inc.

Waldegrave, C., Tamasese, K., Tuhaka, F., and Campbell, W. (2003) *Just Therapy: A Journey. A Collection of Papers From the Just Therapy Team, New Zealand*. Adelaide, SA: Dulwich Centre Publications.

6

WORKING WITH ADDICTIVE BEHAVIOR

Liana Buccieri

Introduction

The following chapter is focused on applying the liberation health approach to working with people struggling with addictive behavior issues. The clinical work presented here was set in a for-profit outpatient mental health clinic in a diverse urban neighborhood. This clinic houses many different programs, including an outpatient addictions treatment program. I worked as a clinician in this addictions treatment program for several years, and it is the context in which I worked with the client described here.

Literature review

Addiction issues in our society can be viewed as symptoms of much larger, systemic problems and the continual effects of these systemic problems on individual people and community groups. The dominant cultural world view dictates that addiction issues be seen as personal problems. Through many venues, this world view is most often unconsciously reinforced. As we see in earlier chapters, a crucial component of liberation health social work is educating about and understanding the dominant cultural world view. In this approach to social work, clinicians and clients collectively work to deconstruct and analyze the oppressive impacts of the dominant worldview on individual clients and communities (Belkin–Martinez 2004). This framework is especially important to integrate within the field of addictive behaviors. While taking responsibility for each of our actions and choices is necessary for growth, externalizing and deconstructing conversations are a crucial way to reduce the blame on individuals and encourage people to actively take control over the problems they see in their lives.

When working with people who misuse substances or have a history of other addictive behaviors, addressing stigmatization, shame, and self-concept is especially important. Negative dominant cultural messages, stereotypes and judgments about "addicts" are pervasive in our society. In the traditional medical model of treatment, most often guiding substance abuse treatment programs, the addiction, the "problem," is always located within the individual. With this approach, addiction is viewed as a disease, and it is the person seeking help who is "sick" with no emphasis in most treatment programs on the sicknesses abundant in the social environment in which we live every day.

An alternative theoretical basis for addictions treatment is offered in psychiatrist Lance Dodes' (2002) *The Heart of Addiction*. While not a liberation health worker, he made a significant contribution to the field of addictions treatment by changing perceptions of why people compulsively do addictive behavior. Dodes' thesis in his book is:

> Virtually every addictive act is preceded by a feeling of helplessness or powerlessness. Addictive behavior functions to repair this underlying feeling of helplessness. It is able to do this because taking the addictive action (or even deciding to take this action) creates a sense of being empowered, of regaining control over one's emotional experience and one's life.
>
> (Dodes 2002: 4)

While he focuses solely on personal problems in people's lives as sources of their feelings of powerlessness, Dodes' theory shares with liberation health an emphasis on the importance of becoming active subjects in our own lives and experiences. As he states:

> The experience of these people underlines the fact that acting in some form when one is trapped and helpless is not only normal, it is psychologically essential. And attempting to act against powerful feelings of helplessness is just what lies at the heart of addiction.
>
> (Dodes 2002: 22)

The harm reduction approach is a model that is extremely client-centered, strengths-based and focused on clients' interpretations of their situations. Together with the liberation health approach, theories of harm reduction are focused on the practice of client empowerment within the therapeutic relationship. With this approach the clients' realities, goals and perspectives on their lives should always be at the forefront of treatment (MacMaster 2004).

A harm reduction approach emphasizes the client's expertise in his/her own life and honors what the client wants to do. Harm reduction, for the sheer fact that it focuses on meeting people where they are in their relationship with addictive behaviors and within the context of other mediating factors, complements and reinforces empowerment-based social work approaches (MacMaster 2004). It also respects that abstinence may not be necessary for every person who has struggled with addictive behavior, and that it is important to collaborate to work towards a client's personal goals rather than prioritizing the clinician's values and ideas of what the client "should" be working on.

In Bernadette Pauly's (2008) article, "Harm reduction through a social justice lens," the author speaks to inequities in health care, focusing on addictions treatment, among homeless or street-involved populations. She speaks to the issue of healthcare access as a major determinant of health, and details the many barriers that exist in accessing comprehensive health care for homeless or low-income, drug-using populations. The perceived stigma and discrimination associated with drug use can negatively impact access to care and the quality of interventions within healthcare settings. Pauly emphasizes the importance of harm reduction programs adopting a "value neutral" approach to drug use and "shifts the moral context in healthcare away from the primary goal of fixing individuals towards one of reducing harm" (Pauly 2008: 6). She notes that the harm reduction approach traditionally emphasizes personal responsibility, and does not address the root socio-political causes contributing to addictive behaviors. Similar to liberation health practice, Pauly goes on to deconstruct concepts of justice in healthcare and encourages increased analysis of the harm created by policies and institutional factors that impact problematic substance use (Pauly 2008).

Addictions treatment has been a rapidly growing industry since the 1990s, and many programs and treatment centers are very expensive and profit-driven. (Morell 1996). In Christopher Smith's (2012) thought-provoking article, "Harm reduction as anarchist practice," he describes the mutually reinforcing relationship between capitalism and addiction. This connection is demonstrated in looking at many structural factors, including the profit-driven nature of the addiction treatment industry, as well as the economic interests of both the illegal drug trade and the business of alcohol manufacturers in encouraging people to remain dependent on the substances they are selling. Smith speaks to the origins of harm reduction work as an illegal, rebellious activity "where activists and politicized front-line workers risked arrest by distributing clean syringes" (p. 210). He goes on to detail the ways that the harm reduction movement has transformed from grassroots political activism, becoming institutionalized within corporate healthcare settings, changing some of the inherent values of the work. The public health policies of harm reduction dictated by government and capitalism "avoid confronting the very things that produce the most harm for drug users: drug laws, dominant discourses of drug use and the stigmatization of users." (p. 211). He encourages a radical critique of the "social and legal systems that create harm" (p. 217) and a confrontation of capitalism's role in producing addiction on a mass scale.

The dominant medical model and Twelve Steps-based treatment programs view the root cause of addiction as illness within each individual. Almost always in these programs, the cultural and institutional factors contributing to addictive behavior remain unaddressed. However, the origins of Alcoholics Anonymous and the Twelve Steps is a grassroots movement, and they continue to operate solely on donations from community members and peers in the recovery community. This community-based foundation complements the liberation health perspective, as Twelve Steps is an approach based in solidarity and collective support. It is a movement of peer-run community groups that are not funded by outside sources, and therefore, are collectively "owned" by the very people who seek help from this form of treatment. In addition, predominantly, throughout its history, the Twelve Steps tradition is a spiritual philosophy to treating addiction, not a medicalized one (Kurtz 1991).

In her article "Radicalizing recovery," Carolyn Morell (1996) introduces another radical analysis into the field of addictions treatment. She offers critical questions and attempts to integrate traditional recovery models (the fellowship of Alcoholics Anonymous and Twelve Steps-based treatment programs) with radical social work methods. Morell speaks to the spiritual aspects of the Twelve Steps model and the opportunities for radical social workers within the addictions field to "blend the liberating aspects of both worldviews (spiritual and political) to promote individual and social change" (Morell 1996: 307). She asserts that the concept of interconnectedness bridges the Twelve Steps recovery and social justice frameworks, and that this core belief motivates both radical socio-political movements and spiritual-based recovery movements. "Divided, people suffer individually and collectively as they experience personal separation and oppression, both of which relate to addictive behavior." (p. 307).

As referenced earlier, self-help recovery groups and group therapy within Twelve Steps-based treatment programs provide settings which reduce the isolation that can fuel and reinforce addictive behaviors. The peer support and solidarity within these environments challenge the cultural message that one is alone with his/her struggles, in both experiencing addiction and in working on recovery. However, in these models, "action" on a socio-political level is seen as taking focus away from work on the individual's behavior change and acceptance of his/her disease of addiction. The focus is predominantly on personal, individual solutions and letting go of control and the need to take action. (Morell 1996).

Morell adds to her analysis of the recovery movement and radical social work by challenging social workers working in recovery group settings to integrate consciousness-raising, political analysis and social action into these contexts. She references innovative recovery programs, such as the Glide Memorial Church program founded by Reverend Cecil Williams in the 1980s in a poor San Francisco neighborhood, which combined individual healing and collective social change (Morell 1996: 310). As Paulo Freire taught, this is the core foundation of liberation health work: the dialectical, consciousness-raising process of changing people internally so that they can act to change the world, as well as changing external conditions so that people can alter their internal experience of the world (Freire 1970). With liberation health work and addictive behaviors, the hope is that people who seek to either end or decrease their dependence on these behaviors, will find other, more powerful actions they can take, such as direct action, organizing and building community solidarity. These may increase self-esteem and connection as well as support change in oppressive conditions.

Romley, Cohen, Ringel, and Sturm (2007) conducted a study entitled "Alcohol and environmental justice," using census data to illustrate the density of liquor stores and bars that people encounter according to race, economic status, and age in various urban areas in the United States. Their results found that the number of liquor stores is far greater in lower-income areas and among non-whites, who more often reside in the lower-income sections of cities across the country. In looking at health disparities and risks across racial/ethnic groups and income groups, the paper addressed the level of "toxicity" within neighborhoods, related to environmental factors. I describe in this chapter these issues that directly relate to the case.

Classism, the cultural and institutional discrimination and oppression of the poor and working class, is a major theme and crucial factor in the case I present here. In legendary feminist author bell hooks' reflection on class, *Where We Stand: Class Matters*, she writes, "Racial solidarity, particularly the solidarity of whiteness, has historically always been used to obscure class, to make the white poor see their interests as one with the world of white privilege" (hooks 2000). As we consider Sean's case in this chapter, there are complex issues of class and race in his story. Sean and I tried to confront exactly what hooks describes about obscuring classism in poor, white communities.

Case summary

Identifying information

Sean is a 47-year-old, white, straight-identified, Irish-American male. He is currently unemployed and living in a transitional housing program for homeless men with a history of addictive behavior.

Referral and presenting problem

Sean was referred to our outpatient clinic for treatment of longstanding "depression and anger issues." The referral source, his case manager at the housing program, also identified these issues in the context of his history of addiction, and noted he was in early sobriety and needed to continue to work on his recovery from addiction.

Course of service

Sean and I met for weekly individual therapy sessions in an urban, outpatient mental health clinic setting for a period of 14 months. The following discussion was written after these 14 months of treatment.

Current situation

Sean came to our first session after eight months of ongoing sobriety and six months into this structured transitional housing program. At the initial meeting, he expressed ambivalence about therapy. Asking for help and speaking about his feelings were very uncomfortable for Sean, and he was skeptical about the helpfulness of treatment. At the same time, after eight months of sobriety, he demonstrated motivation for change. He had gained confidence in his ability to sustain behavior changes through his period of recovery, and given his six months in structured transitional housing, his environment was more familiar and his living situation more stable. Yet, he agreed with his case manager that "I explode too quickly" and that his anger often felt unmanageable and "out of control" once it was triggered. Now that he had been sober for a significant period, Sean felt he needed to address his aggression as it historically had caused problems for him in relationships and jobs, as well as self-injury.

Early on in our sessions, he was able to identify feeling triggered by personal insults, which he began to talk about as "injustices" or "disrespect." He had grown up believing he had to fight back to protect himself, and also to protect "anyone I see as vulnerable; I can never let it go if I see someone picking on the little guy." This sense of moral responsibility and justice often led to behaviors that harmed Sean; it also would prove to be very useful as a foundation in our work together to begin to connect his personal struggles to larger, community level oppression.

In contrast to his explosive behavior, at other times Sean described feeling "very down and like I can't keep going." As we began to talk more about this feeling, he expressed that he felt "stuck" and was unsure what he could do to substantially change how he was feeling. Sometimes, this hopelessness and frustration would manifest outwardly in explosive behavior, and sometimes he internalized it by harming himself, with drugs and alcohol or increased feelings of depression, shame, and self-blame. As we further explored these feelings, we began to understand the core of the problems that Sean experienced (depression, explosive outbursts, addictions) as chronic feelings of isolation and disconnection.

Individual and family history

Sean grew up in an urban neighborhood composed primarily of Irish immigrant families. He was born to first generation Irish-American parents, and was raised with three brothers in a lower-income housing development. His family has a history of alcoholism, and his father drank heavily on a daily basis while Sean was growing up. He witnessed domestic abuse in the home, and was physically and emotionally hurt in his family environment. At the same time, he was raised in a neighborhood where crime and violence were a familiar part of life. Sean began to socialize with a group of aggressive older boys in his early teens. During these years, Sean reports that he witnessed a lot of violence towards non-Irish minorities. He, in turn, learned to fight at an early age and inflicted harm on others to maintain his status in the group. From his early teens, he partook in heavy use of alcohol and drugs. He associated sobriety with vulnerability, because that was when he was consciously aware of feeling scared and hurt. He strongly believed that these feelings were unacceptable and therefore terrifying; he would push them away with drug use and keep up a tough, disaffected image as best he could.

Sean distinctly recalls that his parents did not believe it was acceptable to reach out for help or support from others, even though they struggled to support the family on their own. This history reinforced an engrained belief that one needs to "take care of yourself and pull yourself up" and that expressing vulnerability or asking for support made someone a "weak man and a target" for violence. He acknowledges that he wanted to be feared so people would leave him alone.

Despite having a formal education only through the tenth grade, Sean is extremely intelligent and enjoys learning about a variety of subjects on his own. He expresses that reading is a useful strategy when he is feeling overwhelmed by his own life. He has self-taught carpentry skills, and was a supervisor of construction jobs for many years following high school. He also cared for his ill parents, now deceased, for several years when he was in his late thirties. Although he explains that he had some strong, negative feelings towards his parents related to experiences growing up, he also felt a strong obligation and responsibility as a son to care for them. After both his parents died within a two year span, he became increasingly overwhelmed and his drinking and drug use became heavier. He lost his savings, and eventually became homeless for several years.

Formulation

Sean's story is characterized by chronic feelings of isolation and disconnection. His ongoing struggles with depressive symptoms, aggressive/violent behavior and addictive behavior are shaped by the complex intersection of personal experiences and the social structures, institutions, and cultural practices, class, race, gender, and

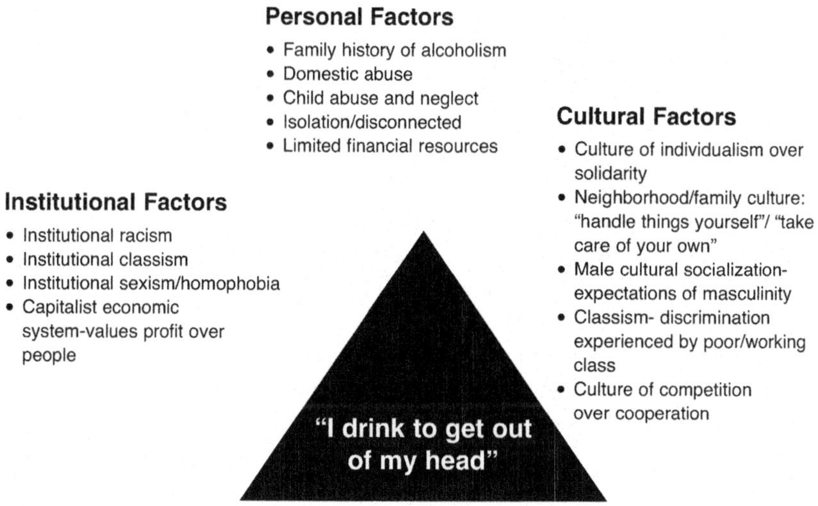

Personal Factors
- Family history of alcoholism
- Domestic abuse
- Child abuse and neglect
- Isolation/disconnected
- Limited financial resources

Cultural Factors
- Culture of individualism over solidarity
- Neighborhood/family culture: "handle things yourself"/ "take care of your own"
- Male cultural socialization-expectations of masculinity
- Classism- discrimination experienced by poor/working class
- Culture of competition over cooperation

Institutional Factors
- Institutional racism
- Institutional classism
- Institutional sexism/homophobia
- Capitalist economic system-values profit over people

"I drink to get out of my head"

FIGURE 6.1 Working with addictive behavior
Source: Liana Buccieri

ethnicity in which he grew up. Addictive behavior, while initially a protective coping strategy for Sean, also served to reinforce further disconnection and isolation from the people around him and the society at large.

In looking at the personal factors that affect Sean, we see an extensive history of trauma in his family. He clearly felt low self-esteem related to the social isolation and violence he experienced and did not feel emotional support from his family as he grew up. Sean's long-standing family history of alcoholism and his own struggle with addiction, may be partially the result of a genetic predisposition for this issue.

On a cultural level, the dominant messages about the value of individualism significantly affected Sean. From his family, he internalized the notion of holding things together on one's own, without asking for help. These messages promoted the idea that everyone can, and should, get ahead on his or her own individual merits and discouraged help from anyone who might be considered an outsider. Additionally, Sean grew up in a patriarchal working class Irish community which had clear expectations around gender roles. He internalized messages around hard, aggressive masculinity in which fighting and drinking were hallmarks of manhood. Again, it was considered unacceptable and weak to seek help from others; if you needed help there was something very wrong with you. Finally, the messages Sean received around race also affected him. His Irish community felt they needed to protect their neighborhood from "outsiders" and influenced the hostility he grew up feeling toward members of other ethnic and racial groups.

Institutional factors impacting Sean's experience of the world are significant contributors to his problems. The definition of environmental injustice includes all factors that compromise a healthy lifestyle, such as the accessibility of excess alcohol in a concentrated area. This accessibility is coupled with limited employment options, poor school systems in urban areas like Sean's, and an illegal drug trade which increases crime and violence in the neighborhood. All of these elements make it very difficult to avoid drug and alcohol use or find legal options to make a living wage to support oneself.

A capitalist economic system that priorities wealth and profit over people's needs thrives on individuals remaining isolated and disconnected from one another. It benefits a capitalist system for similarly oppressed groups to struggle against each other, seeing their "competition" as other poor ethnic groups, all the while distracting them from focusing on the system itself; a system that does not provide a living wage, decent healthcare and affordable housing. This economic system harmed Sean's family and kept them constantly isolated, disconnected and overwhelmed. The intersectionality of these personal, cultural, and institutional factors had a direct impact on Sean's presenting problem and ongoing struggles.

Interventions

Liberation health methodology is rooted in first helping the people we work with to "see the problem" clearly; to identify their individual struggles and experiences in their own words. During this stage, it is very important for social workers to help validate and affirm the person's experience of the world. As people begin to feel supported and validated, this often allows us to begin to work together to analyze people's problems and experiences. In the case of Sean, he had not grown up with any lasting experiences of supportive, growth-producing relationships; he expressed that feeling validated and affirmed in the therapy relationship was a new way of feeling in a relationship.

When I met Sean, he felt a deeply engrained sense of self-blame and shame associated with the chronic disconnections in his life, and these feelings were reinforced by his addictive behaviors throughout his life. Early in our work together, I taught Sean how to draw and analyze a problem tree, a Freirian intervention, which allowed him to identify the effects of addiction on his life, and to deconstruct the root causes of his addictive behavior, on the personal, cultural and institutional levels. Through this consciousness-raising process, he was able to have some compassion for himself seeing his problems as rooted largely outside of him and impacted by so many contributing factors that they were not his fault. He was able to start to think about his life differently and what could be possible for him. We discussed his dialectical feelings of both wanting things to change and to feel better, but also being skeptical and unable to imagine a different way of being. He had never really questioned what he grew up to believe was true about himself and the world, and our initial discussions really shook these automatic beliefs to the core. For Sean, this transformation started with experiencing his ability to connect with another person genuinely and in a way that had a positive impact on both of us.

In efforts to raise "critical consciousness," it is important to help people to deconstruct the dominant worldview assumptions and cultural messages that easily become engrained throughout our lives. In Sean's case, one especially powerful cultural message that pervaded his family and community culture growing up was the myth of individualism that the US capitalist economic system perpetuates. In Sean's neighborhood, most people his family knew did not ask for help when they were struggling, and he did not see many exceptions to the dominant, cultural message that individuals should "take care of yourself and handle your personal business on your own." Early in our sessions, Sean was able to voice his struggle with reconciling these strongly held beliefs with a genuine caring for others and desire to connect, although this was something he fought against in order to protect himself.

In deconstructing these cultural messages about individualism, at the same time that we explored his feelings about his struggles with drug use and mental health concerns, I asked Sean, "Who benefits from your blaming yourself? If it's your fault if you can't pull yourself up on your own, what does that mean for all of us?" We continued to deconstruct the institutional factors, and discussed what it means to live in a capitalist economy and who benefits the most from this economic system. He remarked that he always assumed this economic system worked for him, and benefited him, and wondered aloud how these messages are perpetuated. He brought up the thought that immigrants and other minorities were viewed as "enemies" in his neighborhood growing up, and that there was often talk of "others" stealing the Irish community's jobs. When he broached this, we discussed where those cultural messages come from and, again, whom they really benefit. I posed the idea that maybe it was a distraction from the larger system that was not working for anyone but the most privileged, and this seemed to resonate with him. We explored this idea a bit more, the complexity of racial dynamics in poor communities, and he recognized that he couldn't say why he didn't like these non-white people, except that these assumptions and stereotypes had been engrained in him from a very young age.

I then asked, "What would it be like if your problem, or mine, or anyone's, was considered all of our problem? Our entire community?" I remember him thinking deeply about this for a long while, and eventually saying, "That's crazy. No one would think that, because then someone else is responsible, and it should be my responsibility. These are my problems. If they're not mine, then things really have to change. No one in charge really wants that."

I responded, "That's true, if we're thinking about personal problems this way, that society would need to take on more responsibility for how all of us manage. What does it threaten, then, if we don't see our problems as within individual people?" – "Everything." At that, he laughed and smiled, and I felt a crucial shift in how we were able to talk about his experience.

Relatedly, Sean and I have done a lot of work together challenging cultural messaging about masculinity in his community and in American society at large. We spoke about the ways that these expectations of what it means to be a "real" man have impacted and often harmed Sean throughout his life. When we were exploring his aggressive and explosive behavior, Sean said "I get angry all the time, but I don't know why ... I'm angry at the way things are, but I always thought I needed to suck it up and deal with it ... there was something wrong with me if I couldn't make it on my own." Over time, he was able to identify the way that his deeply held beliefs that men did not express their feelings or show vulnerability or ask for help contributed to his using the more socially acceptable coping strategy of numbing feelings with drugs and alcohol or being violent and expressing anger (the only emotion he grew up believing was acceptable for men to strongly express).

As Sean made connections between his personal issues and cultural factors, we continued to look deeper at where these messages come from in society. Again, the question we came to together was, "Whom do these cultural messages benefit? Why did they develop in the first place?" I asked Sean, "Are they helpful to individual men? Were they helpful to you?" He replied, " You know, I never really thought about it like that. I thought that it helped me to be like that [a hard, aggressive male persona] because I didn't have to deal with anything going on with me, with my family. I could be numb or take it out on people. And for awhile, that helped me deal." We spoke about numbness and apathy and misdirected anger all benefiting the status quo. We spoke about the fact that people who are numb and not allowing themselves to feel their anger or their sadness are not going to try to challenge the way things are. People using drugs and alcohol and so many other forms of addictive behavior to cope with daily struggles helps a dysfunctional economic system that isn't really working for anyone remain in place, unthreatened.

The conversations I was able to have with Sean deconstructing cultural messages demonstrated a pivotal shift in Sean's perspective of his own life and struggles. We began to link his individual symptoms and behaviors more and more to systemic issues; he began to think about the ways that capitalism, classism, racism, and sexism all impacted his struggles and experience in life. We spent a lot of time together working to strengthen Sean's ability to think of himself as someone who is empowered and can be a more active subject in his own life. He is able to think of moments in his life when he has felt empowered to make changes, such as when he started the hard work of staying sober, but "it's hard to feel like you can really change things when you're just one person." We continued to discuss what people can do individually; for instance, in having discussions with other people, to raise consciousness, the way that we have this dialogue about these issues in our time together.

When Sean mentioned being very frustrated by a policy at the shelter where he lived, I asked him if he knew of any other residents who felt similarly. He said that he did not talk to people much, but thought some other men he knew were frustrated too. That week, I asked Sean to think about whether it might be helpful to build some solidarity with other residents of the shelter around this issue; maybe together they would have a greater ability to challenge the policy and advocate for themselves. He agreed that there could be "strength in numbers."

At the time we began to have these discussions, there was a powerful example of community organizing and consciousness raising going on across America through the grassroots Occupy movement. By talking about the work being done by the people involved in this movement, we were able to acknowledge a critical moment for rescuing the historical memory of change in this country. People were coming together to take action around their beliefs about what is right and the world they want to see. That time in our history, and the timing of these conversations with Sean, served as an enormous challenge to the pervasive dominant worldview messaging that there is nothing anyone can do to change the status quo.

Reflections

As I reflect on my experience working with Sean, it is clear to me that we both were changed by the work we did together in our therapeutic relationship. While we were in different roles in this shared clinical experience, at varying stages in our own consciousness-raising processes, and coming from very different places upon meeting, we connected in our efforts to improve his experience of the world. Even though the focus of our work together was clearly on what Sean was feeling and experiencing, it was essential that the relationship between us be growth-producing for both of us if it was going to be for him.

With Sean, I learned more about a world I did not grow up in, and the pressures he faced as a working class Irish-American man in his neighborhood. He taught me about strength, resilience, and the many ways that people find to manage and cope with traumatic experiences in life, and doing what you can do to survive against the odds. As is the case with many people I have worked with, Sean reminded me how quickly people blame themselves for circumstances caused by social and institutional injustices and the immense toll that this takes on the human spirit. I felt the enormity of the pain that can be inflicted upon people by other people, most often in reaction to powerful cultural messaging and institutional deficits. And with him, I also witnessed the incredible capacity that human beings have for hope and change, which clearly was present in even his early efforts to seek out and commit to treatment when he could not yet see any benefits. The vulnerability and openness that he was able to share in exploring some really hard questions and truths about himself and the world inspired me to be braver in this work as well.

I believe deconstructing conversations like the ones I describe above with Sean are the heart of liberation health social work. These are the exciting, pivotal moments in our work when deeply held perceptions and "truths" dictated by the dominant worldview, ones that people may have never been in a position to challenge before, begin to shift. I see so clearly working with Sean that this deconstructing and remembering work can lead to a new vision for his future as an empowered, active subject, rather than a person who experiences the world strictly as an object being acted upon by cultural and institutional systems. As people's views of themselves and the systems at work around them shift, so do their perceptions of what is possible. Liberation health work at its heart is incredibly hopeful and inspiring, which is one of the reasons I am most drawn to it as a clinical practice approach.

In doing this deconstructing, reflecting, and analyzing work with clients, I have seen the ways that people like Sean can come to realize that their personal struggles, whether with addictive behaviors or depressive thinking or aggressive behavior, are not reflective of their worth as human beings. We are all so much more than our problems, and there is not something wrong with us as people if we struggle with addictions or other issues; there are many reasons why the systemic and cultural factors that impact all of us make functioning well within this economic system incredibly difficult, I would argue, for everyone.

The connection between client and therapist as co-collaborators in this work as well as the connection of that relationship to larger community-wide struggles is what can be so powerful. What is most exciting for me about this work is that I always feel that my most often individual, clinical work with clients is connected to something larger, a larger purpose and responsibility as a radical social worker rooted in a social justice perspective. In the same way that I see liberation health work transform and empower my clients' realities, I feel sustained and connected even while working in an office in a clinic.

In thinking about whose interests are served through the mental health system, it is true that most therapists and social workers are trained to help people function better within the existing capitalist system, which is inherently racist, classist, sexist, and heterosexist. We are rarely trained to encourage any questioning of the dominant worldview about the system we all live and work in. The dominant worldview within social work training does not value challenging and deconstructing our realities with our clients. Instead, because the systems of therapy and social work exist within capitalism, there is unconscious value in people being kept isolated and less powerful in order for this economic system to survive. Therefore, one of the most important responsibilities we have as social workers is to speak up when we can to challenge the embeddedness of the dominant worldview in our lives and the system that perpetuates these values. If we don't say anything about this when we are with people, we are silently agreeing with the status quo that the way the system works is acceptable and should not be challenged.

Referring back to Sean's case and the most pivotal consciousness-raising discussion we had, "who benefits from the problems he struggles with being 'his fault'?" Who or what does it threaten if we don't locate problems within people? As I posed to Sean in our session, "What would it be like if 'his' problems were all our problems? What could it be like if this were the framework we lived in?" A major challenge is the consciousness raising work with those who benefit most, with privilege, from the way society is currently structured. We need to transform the dominant cultural worldview about what a truly just social and economic system could be like. We all pay a price when we live in a world that ignores oppression, isolates us from each other and keeps us feeling powerless and hopeless. This system has countless consequences on our communities, our families, and each of us individually. I hope for a world where we collectively prioritize the values of community, solidarity and liberation.

References

Belkin-Martinez, D. (2004) Therapy for liberation: the Paulo Freire methodology. Available online at http://liberationhealth.org/documents/freiresummarysimmons.pdf (accessed October 4, 2013).

Dodes, L. (2002) *The Heart of Addiction*. New York: Harper Collins.

Freire, P. (1970) *Pedagogy of the Oppressed*. New York: Continuum.

hooks, b. (2000) *Where We Stand: Class Matters*. New York: Routledge.

Kurtz, E. (1991) *Not-god: A History of Alcoholics Anonymous*. Center City, MN: Hazelden Educational Materials.

MacMaster, S. (2004) Harm reduction: a new perspective on substance abuse services. *Social Work*, 49 (3): 356–63.

Morell, C. (1996) Radicalizing recovery: Addiction, spirituality and politics. *Social Work*, 41 (3): 306–12.

Pauly, B. (2008) Harm reduction through a social justice lens. *International Journal of Drug Policy*, 19 (1): 4–10.

Romley, J.A., Cohen, D., Ringel, J., and Sturm, R. (2007) Alcohol and environmental justice: The density of liquor stores and bars in urban neighborhoods in the United States. *Journal of Studies on Alcohol and Drugs*, 68 (1): 48–55.

Smith, C. B. R. (2012) Harm reduction as anarchist practice: A user's guide to capitalism and addiction in North America. *Critical Public Health*, 22 (2): 209–21.

7

WORKING WITH AFRICAN-AMERICANS

Johnnie Hamilton-Mason

This chapter describes work with a woman of African descent who is a psycho-therapy client at an urban community health center. As is usually true, the one descriptor, "of African descent," is a crucial and incomplete descriptor. This parti-cular woman is also an immigrant, highly educated, professional and married. The chapter attends particularly to our work together as it relates to her, and my, African descent.

I hope to demonstrate how the liberation health model may be used to formulate, assess, and intervene with my client, who identifies as African-American. I focus on historical legacy, kinship, collectivism and the way that she sees and understands her life. I discuss and highlight aspects of our work that contribute to her emerging critical consciousness, liberation, collectivism and political activism to respond to the stressors that brought her to therapy.

Setting and population

Behavioral health services at the Community Health Center aims to provide quality care to adult and child consumers who are chronically mentally ill and who may be experiencing moderate to severe emotional, developmental, and environ-mental difficulties. The services include individual counseling, group counseling, family counseling, couples therapy, and psychiatric consultation. Many clinicians are bilingual in Spanish. The services to children are both clinic-based and school-based, with school-based services provided at some public schools. Additionally, the Center provides community based services for the Department of Mental Health. The inner-city population served at the clinic is multi-racial, multi-ethnic and predominately low income. The writer is an African-American social worker who provides therapy at the Center. The client, whom I will call Andrea, belongs to four intersecting identities, often in subordinate positions in our society: African descent, immigrant, female, and mentally ill. At the same time, she is well educated and has stable employment, housing and income and most would consider her privileged.

Population demographics

African-Americans comprise 12.7 percent of the total US population. Females head 28 percent of African-American households, which is more than double the national figure of 12.6 percent female-headed households (US Census 2011). Unemployment rates for African-Americans are higher than national figures (16.7 percent of African-Americans vs. 10.3 percent of the general population) and 21.2 percent of African-American men and 12.8 percent of African-American women are unemployed. 80.2 percent of American-Americans have less than a bachelor's degree; while national numbers report 70.1 percent of individuals possess less than a bachelor's degree (US Bureau of the Census 2011).

Literature review

This literature review is organized to underscore the conceptual and empirical literature most relevant to Andrea and her family, ultimately addressing essential characteristics of African-American families. The following areas are included: historical legacy, family resilience, black feminist thought, post colonialism and liberation health. All the literature emphasizes socio-cultural factors and resistance.

Historical legacy

Collectivism is the thread that ties together all of the streams of conceptual and empirical literature discussed in this section. There are three premises that are critical to understanding collectivism among African-Americans; individual identity is a collective identity, the spiritual aspect of humans is the essence of human existence; and the affective approach to knowledge is epistemologically valid (Harvey 2001).

Collectivism, in contrast to individualism, emphasizes embeddedness of individuals in a larger group. African culture, which informs the world view of African-Americans, is characterized by themes of unity and harmony, of wholeness and equilibrium (Ani 2004; Billingsley and Caldwell 1994). An African cultural paradigm considers "the needs of the group first, believing that in so doing, individual needs and desires will be met" (Nobles 1986: 35). This overarching way of relating to the world contributes to adaptability and resistance with African-Americans. From the perspective of liberation psychology, "there is no person without family, no learning without culture, no madness without social order; and therefore neither can there be an I without a we, a knowing without a symbolic system" (Martín-Baró 1994: 41).

Long before Africans were brought to the United States and elsewhere as slaves, they descended from ancient civilizations on the continent of Africa that viewed family and kin as a precondition for success. Historically, African culture's collectivist world view influenced its philosophical, political and, religious orientation. John Mbiti (1990) underscores the important sense of the community among traditional Africans. In traditional Africa, the individual does not and cannot exist alone, except physically. Africans owe their existence to other people, including those of past generations as well as contemporaries. Marimba Ani states "Africa survives in our spiritual make up; that is the strength and depth of African spirituality and humanism that has allowed for the survival of African-Americans as a distinctive cultural entity in America" (Ani 2004: 1).

Family resilience

How their ancestors adapted to enormous upheavals and social dislocation experienced during and after slavery continues to influence how African-Americans manage their everyday lives. Andrew Billingsley asserts that the African-American family is "an intimate association of persons who are related to one another by a variety of means, including blood, marriage, formal adoption, informal adoption, or by appropriation" (Billingsley 1992: 28). He also maintains that African-American families are sustained by a history of resilience in America, and are deeply embedded in a network of social structures both internal and external to themselves (Billingsley 1992). Scholars have documented the presence of stable resilience (Ani 2004; Billingsley 1992; Boyd-Franklin 2010; Nobles 1986: Mbiti 1990), asserting that these enduring characteristics of survival and adaptability contribute to strengths of African-Americans today. Previous generations of scholars focused on deviation and weakness, more often using the Western culture's acceptance of the "model" nuclear family as their definition of family; whereas recently, other theorists have documented the resourcefulness, adaptability and resilience of the black family. For example, Andrew Billingsley asserts "if black families were in trouble, it was not some inherent, cultural condition which was at the heart of deterioration, but socioeconomic factors pressing in from outside" (Billingsley 1992: 11).

Many studies have found family to be a significant component of resilience, although they qualify and describe its influence in different ways (Bell-Tolliver, Burgess and Brock 2009; Carter-Black 2001; Davis 2007; Murphy 2009). Several studies find religion to be another common theme among resilient people (Bell-Tolliver, Burgess, and Brock 2009; Carter-Black 2001; Davis 2007).

Spirituality and the black church

Throughout history, particularly during slavery, people of African descent have held strong spiritual and religious beliefs. They had to be spiritual beings and in touch with their spiritual selves to survive hate, racism, and sexism (Mattis 2002; Starks and Hughey 2003). Spirituality continues to be a strong influence on and an important factor among African-Americans (Boyd-Franklin 2010; Mattis 2002;

Mbiti 1990; Starks and Hughey 2003). Traditionally, religion and religious institutions, namely the black church, have been recognized as fundamental elements in the spiritual lives of many black Americans (Billingsley 1992; Boyd Franklin 2010). Data from the US Religious Landscape Survey document that 78 percent of black Americans identify as Protestant and three in four black Protestants indicate their affiliation with a historically black church (Pew Forum 2009). The black church provides both a theological and sociocultural perspective from which to address the complex stressors many black women face (Taylor, Chatters, and Levin 2004). In addition to the religious teachings, the black church also provides important social supports (Boyd-Franklin 2010). Some of these include tangible aid; political and social advocacy; and a range of community programming such as financial literacy training, youth development activities, health initiatives, and marriage enrichment programs (Lewis and Truelar 2008; Taylor *et al.* 2004).

Research suggests that black women are more likely than men to hold membership in religious institutions, attend worship services more regularly, and engage in private acts of devotion more frequently (Mattis 2002). According to the US Religious Landscape Survey (Pew Forum 2009), 84 percent of African-American women say that religion is very important to them, and 59 percent report attendance at religious services at least once a week. Further, 62 percent of African-American women report membership within a historically black Protestant church (Pew Forum 2009). It is important to note that, although religion and spirituality are different, in black culture they may be viewed as inseparable because during slavery, and afterwards this was the only institution that was allowed to flourish with and without the sanctions of their oppressors. In fact, this was the core arena where African-Americans used collective resistance strategies against their oppressors.

For African-American women more than for black men, spirituality remains a way of negotiating and making meaning about the issues, struggles and forms of oppression that they face in their everyday lives (Mattis 2002). In contrast to many others for whom the psychological and spiritual domains are separate, the African belief system suggests that the psyches and the spiritual are one (Mbiti 1990; Nobles 1986).

In spite of the contributions to knowledge about the significance of an African-American family's strengths, including strong kinship ties and spirituality (Billingsley 1992; Boyd-Franklin 2003; Hill Collins 2000), and resilience (Carter-Black 2001; Murphy 2009; Davis 2007), a gendered and a postcolonial analysis are not usually contained in these discussions. An inclusion of these theoretical lenses broadens practitioners' work from focusing on individual and/or family attributes to a wider examination of how racism, sexism and other structural forces impede true liberation.

Black feminist thought

Black feminist thought consists of theories or specialized thought produced by African-American women, and intended to express a black woman's standpoint

(Hamilton-Mason, Hall, and Everett 2009). Core themes linked to racism, sexism, classism, together with other forms of oppression and what women do to resist, are aspects of this standpoint. Black feminists are attentive to the diversity of black women's experiences in encountering these core themes; the varying expressions of consciousness regarding the core themes and their experiences with them; and the interdependence of black women's experiences, consciousness, and actions (Hill Collins 2000). A core goal of black feminist thought is to empower black women by recognizing how gender, race and class intersect and are socially constructed. Black feminists articulate that liberation of black women entails freedom for all people, since it would require the end of racism, sexism, and class oppression (Hill Collins 2000). Over the years, there has been a critical alliance between postcolonial feminist and black feminist thought (Comas-Diaz, Lykes, and Alarcon 1998; Hill Collins 2000). Both have struggled for recognition, not only from men in their own culture, but also from Western feminists.

The concept of intersectionality, introduced initially by Crenshaw (1989, 1991) and reintroduced by Patricia Hill Collins (2000), is intrinsic to black feminist thought. Intersectionality is a concept referring to the ways in which socially and culturally constructed categories interact on multiple levels to manifest themselves as inequality in society. It posits oppressions based on identity constructs, such as race/ethnicity, gender, religion, nationality, sexual orientation, class, or disability do not act independently of one another; instead, these forms of oppression inter-relate, creating a system of oppression that reflects the "intersection" of multiple forms of discrimination (Hill Collins 2000: 1–20).

Post-colonialism

Post-colonial theory provides a lens with which to understand identity, gender, race, racism, and ethnicity. More specifically, it underscores how knowledge of the world is generated under specific relations between those who have power and those who do not (Fanon 1967). Franz Fanon analyzed the nature of colonialism and those subjugated by it. He describes colonialism as a source of violence rather than a violent reaction against resistors, which had been the common view (Fanon 1963). In fact, he was among the first to discuss the evolution of microagression and internalized oppression. Fanon (1967) states that an integral part of colonialism is the devalorization of the history and culture of colonized people. This will lead to their negative self-perception and self-portrayal. The colonial process promotes a sense of inferiority among the colonized. A post-colonial analysis simultaneously accounts for the current and historical repercussions of oppressive forces, including sexism, racism, homophobia, and classism. (Almeida, Dolan-DelVecchio, and Parker 2007). This analysis recommends that social workers consistently attend to "their clients' diversity of backgrounds; including their communities' experience of oppression and privilege as a fundamental part of the liberation endeavor … it authenticates the intervention process by bringing it in line with the family's longstanding efforts towards cultural resistance and survival" (ibid: 176–7).

Liberation health

Martín-Baró's articulation of a psychology of liberation echoed earlier work by Franz Fanon (1967), liberation theology (Parham 2002; Ani 2004) and the pedagogy of oppression elaborated by Paulo Freire (1967, 1970). It resonates well with work of a number of African-American psychologists and social workers. The goal of liberation is achieved through critical analysis of the particular situations and actions of the popular majority (Martín-Baró, 1994, 1996; Montero 1990). Psychology of liberation focuses on the collective rather than the individual and serves as a vehicle for the satisfaction of human needs (Bulhan 1985). Accordingly, Martín-Baró (1994, 1996) emphasized that "the first step of liberating structures is to address the social structures, followed by the personal or psychological ones ... that maintain a situation of moral oppression of the majority of people" (1994, p. 26). Freedom can only be achieved through political and socio-cultural activism.

Case study

Identifying information and referral

Andrea is a 39-year-old black woman, married to 40-year-old Joseph for the past nine years. The couple has three children: two, aged 22 and 18, are the result of Joseph's first relationship in his home country; the third is a son, aged 5. Andrea graduated from high school and has a bachelor's and a master's degree. She is employed as a high-level administrator in city government. Joseph is self-employed as a construction contractor and manages the couple's rental properties. Andrea was referred to me at an outpatient mental health clinic following a brief hospitalization for suicidal ideation and a diagnosis of an affective illness in 2009.

Current situation

Owing to her recent diagnosis, Andrea was placed on several psychotropic medications to treat a major depression and/or a bipolar disorder. Her chief complaint was: "I was just discharged from a psychiatric hospital and I continue to feel overwhelmed by my life ... I am the main provider for my family and everything has caught up with me. I would be lying to you if I told you I don't still think about killing myself. I don't have a plan and I don't intend to, but it is still there." The other precipitant factors for her inpatient hospitalization included financial stress related to the mortgage crises, and the death of the maternal aunt who helped to raise her in her country of origin. According to Andrea, she has made previous suicide attempts, including taking pills and a large amount of alcohol. She also self-injured (via cutting) in order to "see blood" when she was in college, and she cut her arms once during the beginning of our therapy.

Relevant history

Andrea was born in a Central/Latin American country and is the descendent of African slaves. Her parents separated when she was two years old. At that time, her mother migrated to the United States, leaving Andrea for 12 years to be cared for by her maternal grandmother and aunt. Andrea's mother had two sons in the United States, fathered by another man. Andrea was brought up in a large extended family in the urban capital city of her native country, living below the poverty level. She immigrated to the United States at age 14 in 1988. Joseph, her husband, was born in another Central American country and is also a descendent of African slaves. He immigrated to the United States in 1994.

Andrea graduated from college and received a master's degree. She has been married for nine years and has one biological son and two stepdaughters. Her first language is Spanish; however, she is comfortable speaking both Spanish and English. She perceives her family, especially her husband and children, as supportive. However, her relationship with her mother is experienced as inconsistent and only occasionally supportive.

Andrea is attractive; brown skinned, tall, of medium physique with long natural dreadlocks. She is an engaging, warm, intelligent and witty woman who self-identifies as African-American. She has a group of female friends, and she more recently attends a progressive black church near her home. She has been consistently employed since graduating from college and has had increasing responsibility at work.

Andrea has a history of sexual assault by a cousin at age three and again at 14 years of age by the same cousin, who had followed Andrea shortly after her reunification with her mother, living briefly with the family. In addition to her own sexual trauma, she witnessed, from age 14 until she left home for college at 18, her mother being physically abused by her stepfather. She reports a history of frequent nightmares and sleeping only two or three hours at night, going to bed only after she becomes extremely tired. She has used substances such as alcohol and marijuana at times, but approximately six months prior to her hospitalization she became concerned about her increasing use of alcohol and stopped drinking.

Formulation

It is important to contextualize Andrea's presenting crises based upon a Freirian analysis of personal and family history, cultural and institutional factors (Freire 1967; Belkin-Martinez 2004). The push and pull factors of immigration, transnationalism and capitalism are interrelated aspects of her lived experience. Although there are distinct elements of pain, suffering and struggle, there are also elements of agency and resisting oppression (Moane 2003).

The personal factors affecting Andrea relate to constraints and suffering concerning her vacillating feelings of maternal abandonment and anger about being raped at age three, and again at 14 years of age by an older cousin. She was also mourning the deaths of a loving grandmother and aunt whose physical proximity was limited after her arrival in this country. Subsequent to her reunification with her mother, she witnessed consistent physical and emotional abuse of her mother by the mother's boyfriend who fathered her two younger brothers. At various times since her adolescence, she has experienced flashbacks, sleeplessness, anxiety, and hopelessness, and a general feeling of being "overwhelmed." Andrea has had feelings of inferiority and internalized oppression, in addition to shame, degradation, and powerlessness over her mental health problems. The oppressive boundaries set by race, gender, and class were sometimes overwhelming, but they were also mediated by tremendous personal accomplishments in secondary and post-secondary education, in her marriage and in her professional achievement.

The cultural factors influencing Andrea include her roles as wife, mother, stepmother, and daughter. Cultural influences that impact her day-to-day life relate to her gendered vulnerability, especially the expectations that she has for herself, as well as those expected by others.

Andrea and Joseph have similar and different post-colonial histories; each of their home countries has unique cultures and subcultures developed over centuries of indigenous traditions, as well as colonialism, slavery and struggles for independence (Almeida *et al.* 2007; Fanon 1967; Boyd-Franklin 2010). Many of the same factors directly and indirectly pushed them to migrate to the United States. They both came from hierarchal societies that were stratified based on race, class, and culture. For example, dark-skin people were more devalued within their families and in society. (Almeida *et al.* 2007; Fanon 1967; Cesaire 1972). Combined with these challenges, Andrea faces stressors that many women deal with in addition to racism and classicism. She exists within complex multi-layered shifting cultural, racial contexts that are influenced by traditional gender patterns that include an unjust distribution of labor in her family and marriage.

Additional stressors are related to her experiences of being caught between varied cultural expectations. Andrea struggled with trying to acknowledge family ties to her mother and norms that assign roles according to gender, age, and status, and birth order. As the eldest and female, Andrea was expected to defer to her mother and take care of her mother. There was a blending of different cultures between Andrea and Joseph; while her employment required an ability to shift to dominant (white) cultural norms in order to meet expectations during the day.

The more salient institutional factors influencing Andrea relate to living and working in a mostly segregated urban environment in the northeast. The institutional arrangement of economics, education, health and welfare within a hierarchical, racially and ethnically oppressed urban community fosters her sense of fragmentation and classism. Certainly, her being one of a few black people at work and the only one at her level is an institutional stressor. Workplace policies are another institutional factor. She has excelled in school and apparently found those institutions supportive.

Other institutional factors involve Andrea's country of origin. Geographically situated between South and Central Latin America, it was always influenced by the

United States' interference in economic policy. The political and hierarchical power structure was dominated almost exclusively by a small number of aristocratic families. This largely urban oligarchy tended to be white or light-skinned, and valued its purported racial purity; aristocrats intermarried and held tightly to their elite status. Government was controlled by a small group of people that also controlled the economy, education and health systems. These factors resulted in pushing waves of poor and middle-class families to migrate. Finally, there were similar factors influencing Andrea living and working in a segregated urban environment in the northeast of the United States.

Interventions

The interventions include analyzing the problem, recovering history, deconstructing the messages and introducing new information.

Analyzing the problem

Andrea tended to personalize her problems in the beginning of our work together, saying that she felt alone and inadequate. Through structured dialogue during assessment, we actively explored all of the conditions that contributed to the depression that precipitated her referral, using the Freirean triangle (Belkin-Martinez 2004) as a tool to help broaden her awareness of the sociopolitical factors, and not just the personal ones. Freire defines praxis as "reflection and action upon

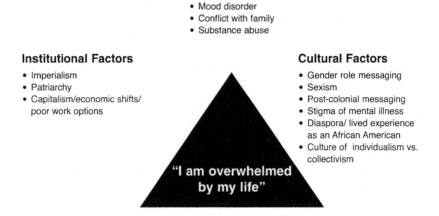

FIGURE 7.1 Liberation health and African-Americans

Source: Johnnie Hamilton-Mason

the world in order to transform it" (Freire 1970: 33). Through praxis, oppressed people can acquire a critical awareness of their own condition, and, with their allies, struggle for liberation. As we collaborated on developing the triangle and listing personal, cultural and institutional factors (see Figure 7.1) that contributed to her feeling so overwhelmed, she reported feeling relieved, and she commented that many of her challenges were outside of her control, which lessened her responsibility and self-blame. As Andrea and I completed the triangle, she gained a different perspective on her problems. Within a couple of weeks after we began working together, Andrea went back to work part time. She continued to feel depleted and stigmatized, because she did not feel she was able to meet all that was expected of her. At this point she described her difficulty in terms of others' expectations, not just her own failure. She talked about feeling "sick and tired of all of the things I have to do as wife, mother, daughter, sister and professional worker."

As I posed questions, and we problem solved, particular patterns and themes emerged. The two most prominent personal themes were Andrea's recounting of her sense of parental abandonment coupled with her feelings of alienation and loss over her maternal grandmother's and aunt's deaths; both had died within months of each other in her home country. Other themes involved the expectations of her as a woman at home and as a representative of her race, and of her gender at work. The structure of her job, which seemed to depend on workers' having wives at home, was also a theme. She noted her sense of difference and isolation in relation to her colleagues and to her local black community, and her shame about her mental illness diagnosis and hospitalization. As she analyzed her experience, her consciousness increased about the root causes of her personal problems related to larger socio-structural and economic factors. It became clearer to Andrea that with the absence of her large extended family that remained in her home country, she was especially lacking family support, as she had a strained relationship with her mother and her two younger brothers.

Setting goals was crucial to our work together. She and I agreed to place her needs related to the sense of alienation from her social and cultural network as an area of prominence. Andrea also agreed to talk to her husband about joining our sessions. She acknowledged that although Joseph tries to be helpful, he is shocked and confused. The interventions were the result of a blending of Andrea's and my perspectives related to the factors and themes we identified together. However, it is important to acknowledge that each step along the way was motivated by Andrea's increasing desire to take actions that she found restorative.

Recovering history

We analyzed Andrea's country of origin's history. I believe that Andrea's ability to dialogue and teach me about her Latin and African influenced culture contributed to our relationship as we engaged in this process. Her world view was shaped by the colonial power structure that devalorized the history of her African and indigenous ancestors. She began to articulate the importance in her culture of the family as the reference point where one's existence is perceived as being interconnected and communal (Billingsley 1992). At the same time, she was able to identify and articulate multiple resistance strategies her people had developed as they survived in a post-colonial country where their access to power was limited (Jones and Shorter-Gooden 2003). This process led to discussions about her pre- and post-immigration experiences. The personal, cultural and institutional dimensions of Andrea's family history were elicited through asking questions about her country of origin, about key family members, identification of family members who were supportive, beliefs about mental and physical health for existing family and past generations, and gender roles within and outside of her family. This process also included obtaining details about the role of spirituality and religion in her life. As she discovered memories of her kinship network's legacy of survival, she became much more aware of their collective struggles against power inequalities in a system which maintained insufficient material resources especially for poorest people more often of African descent.

One similarity shared by African-American, Caribbean, and Latin American families is their African cultural heritage and forced enslavement in countries where they were racially, culturally and linguistically dominated by their captors. As a consequence of exposure to various forms of oppression blacks throughout the diaspora employed physical, psychological, and collective opposition.

Deconstructing the dominant messages

This critical part of our work is illustrated by the following discussion about the community in her home country. The city in which she lived is still described as two cities: the free-trade zone that bustles with global business, and the poverty-stricken outer city, which is still suffering an economic depression. People of African descent were denied access to stable employment within the restricted international part of the city. She began to critique the ways in which class, race, gender and systems of power influenced her conceptions of herself, and how she measured the worth of her family life in her country of origin and in the United States (Hernandez, Almedia and Del Vecchio 2005). She also connected to ways in which economic exploitation, globalization, colonialism, and corrupt government structures contributed to her family's disadvantage.

There are several instances below that are exemplars of the significance of a liberation health analysis for Andrea. During the first occasion, Andrea and I were talking about her former neighborhood, near the Caribbean sea, with collapsing buildings, high unemployment, crime and despair. The infrastructure and economic disparities suffered by the darkest-skinned residents of her former section of the city often led to spontaneous protests in the streets. As she talked about the color caste system of race that exists in her country, she also made the point that within her family and her immediate neighborhood, the color line was also still used as a way to valorize some. The darkest-skinned people suffered more than lighter-skinned people, as they were more stigmatized and often were without formal work needed to support their families. According to Fanon (1967), everything associated with the colonized is portrayed as negative and inferior in comparison to the colonizer. The colonizer should be emulated while the colonized should be despised. Countering these oppressive disempowering mechanisms is the positive cycle of transformation or liberation marked by an increased awareness, social identification of issues, and empowerment to challenge oppressions on personal, relational, and systemic levels (Fanon 1967).

Another example is revealed in the following illustration. Andrea recalled the one-bedroom apartment in which her maternal grandmother lived, caring for her grandchildren and other extended family members. At this time, she also talked about how her mother always sent checks to support her materially, but she felt that her mother never tried to bridge the gap created by their separation emotionally. She described her amazement at how much her grandmother did with so few resources. Her memories of her grandmother were marked by how she also managed to care for her grandchildren and other extended family members with only a first-grade education. Further education had been denied her because she was female and because she was dark skinned, and her family needed her income.

Andrea also strengthened her solidarity with her husband as her deconstruction of information expanded from the plight of women back home and in this country to the role she held in her relationship with her husband. Since Joseph was also included in our meetings every other week, he grew in recognition that he had a part in colluding with unreasonable expectations of Andrea as wife and mother. This aware-ness was the result of a collaborative intervention that involved a power analysis; the three of us deconstructed and critiqued the messages that Andrea and Joseph had learned about gender in their respective countries of origin. This analysis, a series of questions and answers about the role of women, further reinforced awareness of the intergenerational personal, cultural and institutional messages that are learned before we have words for them. As he took on more day-to-day household tasks, such as caring for their young son, transporting him back and forth to school, cooking, and cleaning, he became more aware of how many tasks Andrea performed. Joseph grew in his consciousness of the multiple ways in which women were subjugated and how this contributed to an accumulation of stressors. Joseph also acknowledged the effect that Andrea's mother had on her. Together, they strategized about how to minimize her negative energy while recognizing that Andrea's mother was also subjugated, a survivor of domestic violence, marginalized as a female within her country of origin, as well as in the United States.

According to Ignacio Martín-Baró (1996), we live burdened by the lie of a prevailing discourse that denies, ignores, or disguises essential aspects of reality. As Andrea participated in contextualizing her crises and her family's crises within the larger trials of historical and contemporary racism and sexism that she experienced, we exposed the lies of this discourse, and unveiled a reality that had been denied by prevailing society. Identifying the ways in which colonized and enslaved cultures resisted domination provided a backdrop of liberation for Andrea (Almeida *et al.* 2007: 5).

Introducing new information

One of the most critical interventions for Andrea related to finding a community-based activists' group. She selected a women's group at her church. Prior to her hospitalization, Andrea had infrequently worshipped at an African Methodist church in her community that had been a major gathering place for abolition meetings and rallies prior to the American Civil War, and remained a focal activist congregation. The group is a powerful example of how liberation health principles, based in part upon liberation psychology, are often present in the context of a preexisting resistance group or niche of resistance (Moane 2003, 2011).

Andrea found a place where she came to understand that she was not alone in her personal struggles with being overwhelmed. The group consisted of approximately 15 women, who met weekly to redevelop the church's educational leadership center. Andrea became very involved in this group, as they discussed the ways in which educational equity was important for children in their community, and as they began to appreciate that their best efforts alone were insufficient. They realized they needed to organize with a citywide coalition, and the church group became part of a citywide action network. She began to talk in our meetings about the root causes of educational inequality in our community and to identify similar causes in her home county. The theory and practice of liberation psychology emerges from an oppressed community's expressing the desire to change the status quo, and takes the position that an individual's psychology and their political environment are not only linked, but interact dynamically with each other. Therefore, not only can oppression have negative impacts on health; but also resisting oppression and instigating political change as an act of liberation, can have positive psychological effects (see for instance, Lykes and Moane 2003; Moane 2011).

More importantly, she began to talk about the solidarity she felt towards the less educated community members who, like her grandmother and other relatives, lacked better opportunities. She also understood that her access to education had not protected her from being marginalized as a black woman at her job. Andrea acknowledged that this revelation led to her personal empowerment and solidarity with other members of the community who were unable to attain upward movement. We simultaneously in our individual sessions followed the discourse that began in her group. We also critiqued how the school department reinforces larger society's view of working class and inner city residents who rely on public education.

There was another powerful intervention that took place towards the end of my writing this chapter. Andrea had given me permission to use her work with me as a case example, and I collaborated with her frequently throughout the writing process. I provided her with a draft of the chapter in a recent session, and we discussed her reactions. As we talked she became more and more animated. She began to spontaneously provide more details about her life, especially about her grandmother.

Andrea told me stories about her maternal grandmother, who had talked to her about resisting the devaluing of her identity as indigenous, dark skinned and black. She talked about how her grandmother resisted being stigmatized and told her "marry a black man." As previously mentioned, the colonized can accept or resist the manifestations of their oppression (Fanon 1967) Andrea believed this was a form of resistance, She followed up and sent me a picture of her great grand-mother, who was a very dark-skinned women looking as if she could have been Cherokee and black in the United States, but who identified as black. Moreover, she stressed to Andrea the way out of poverty is education.

Reflections

An essential and overarching theme of our work related to how we were able to explore the parts of our lives that intersected and overlapped as black women. As a result, our work encompassed affective communication about how similar we were. "Many people of African ancestry, whether they use the name African or not have been and continue to be African in behavior maintaining cultural connections and traditions" (Parham 2002: xx). African culture's continuing presence blended with Latin colonial culture as a major component of Andrea's worldview about famil-ismo or collectivism.

I believe that Andrea's ability to dialogue and teach me about her culture and her world view contributed to our relationship, at the same time as it enabled her to engage in problem-solving actions. It became enormously important and challenging for Andrea to give up her assumption that she was the only one who could keep things going for her family. However, her participation in the women's group at her church provided a communal alliance that became an important source of collective, spiritual and relational empowerment. Her women's group became a place and a space where she learned skills by interrogating the economic and political foundations of oppression within her current community.

Recently, Andrea invited me to be on a panel at her church, sponsored by members of the above group. The purpose of the panel was to discuss mental health, black women, and how they cope with stress. In addition to her group, other invited women represented a coalition of groups from various black churches within the metropolitan area. The women meet several times a year as part of a collaborative to share resources and collective power. At the end of the panel's discussion, Andrea got up and revealed to the collective that she has struggled with mental health issues of her own, and she introduced me to the group as her therapist. In doing so, I believe that she was linking the various supports in her life that were previously separate. It is significant to notice that she was willing to take the risk of revealing this information about herself, and making herself vulnerable to the group.

Why was she motivated to do this? I believe it reflects her desire to share with her community and to help other women who might benefit from hearing about her own experiences. She has grown, and become conscious of the factors that have affected her, and wants to raise consciousness in the group. Also, she now has a deeper understanding of how so many of the factors that contributed to her mental health issues were not internal, personal problems, but were actually institutional, cultural, and historical aspects of oppression. She now recognizes that so much of her struggle comes from outside of herself, from oppression due to her gender and race that these women also face. Working collectively with the members of her group, she is helping them see the factors outside themselves that contribute to stress in their lives and their overall mental health.

The process of sharing parts of the chapter with her was in itself an intervention. As a part of the process of reading the draft, she started to talk about her ancestors and shared with me a photograph of her great grandmother. In doing so, she was "rescuing the historical memories" about her ancestors. One of the most important aspects of our relationship began with agreement about the importance of the inextricable cultural link of an African world view operating within people of African descent irrespective of where they were born.

References

Almeida, R., Dolan-Del Vecchio, K., and Parker, L. (2007) Foundation concepts for social justice based therapy: Critical consciousness, accountability, and empowerment. In E. Aldarondo (ed.) *Promoting Social Justice Through Mental Health Practice*. Mahwah, NJ: Lawrence Erlbaum Associates, pp. 175–206.

Ani, M. (2004) *Let the Circle be Unbroken: The Implications of African Spirituality in The Diaspora*. Atlanta, GA: Nkonimfo Publications.

Belkin, Martinez, D. (2004) Therapy for liberation: the Paulo Freire methodology. Available online at http://liberationhealth.org/documents/freiresummarysimmons.pdf (accessed October 4, 2013).

Bell-Tolliver, L., Burgess, R., and Brock, L. J. (2009) African American therapists working with African American families: An exploration of the strengths perspective in treatment. *Journal of Marital and Family Therapy*, 35 (3): 293–307.

Billingsley, A. (1992) *Climbing Jacob's Ladder: The Enduring Legacy of African American Families*. New York: Simon and Schuster.

Billingsley, A. and Caldwell, C. H. (1994) The social relevance of the contemporary Black church. *National Journal of Sociology*, 8 (1–2): 1–24.

Boyd-Franklin, N. (2003) Black families in therapy: The African American experience. New York, NY: Guilford Press.

Boyd-Franklin, N. (2010) Incorporating spirituality and religion into the treatment of African American clients. *The Counseling Psychologist*, 38 (7): 976–1000.

Bulhan, H. (1985) *Frantz Fanon and the Psychology of Oppression*. New York: Plenum.

Carter-Black, J. (2001) The myth of "the tangle of pathology": Resilience strategies employed by middle-class African American families. *Journal Of Family Social Work*, 6 (4): 75–100.

Cesaire, A. (1972) *Discourse on Colonialism*. New York: Monthly Review Press.

Comas-Díaz, L., Lykes, M. B., and Alarcón, R. D. (1998) Ethnic conflict and the psychology of liberation in Guatemala, Peru, and Puerto Rico. *American Psychologist*, 53: 778–92.

Crenshaw, K. (1989) Demarginalizing the intersection of race and sex: A Black feminist critique of antidiscrimination doctrine, feminist theory and antiracist politics. *University of Chicago Legal Forum*, 139–67.

Crenshaw, K.W. (1991) Mapping the margins: Intersectionality, identity politics, and violence against women of color. *Stanford Law Review*, 43 (6): 1241–99.

Davis, J. L. (2007) An Exploration of the Impact of Family on the Achievement of African American Gifted Learners Originating from Low-income Environments. (Unpublished doctoral dissertation). Williamsburg, VA: College of William and Mary.

Fanon, F. (1963) *The Wretched of the Earth*. New York: Grove Press.

Fanon, F. (1967) *Black Skin, White Masks*. Trans. C. L. Markmann. New York: Grove Weidenfeld.

Freire, P. (1967) *Education as the Practice of Freedom in Education for Critical Consciousness*. New York: Continuum.

Freire, P. (1970) *Pedagogy of the Oppressed*. New York: Continuum.

Hamilton-Mason, J., Hall, J. C., and Everett, J. (2009) And some of us are braver: Stress and coping among African American women 18–55 years of age. *Journal of Human Behavior in the Social Environment*, 19 (5): 463–82.

Harvey, A. (2001) Individual and family intervention skills with African Americans: An afrocentric approach. In R. Fong and S. Furuto (eds), *Culturally Competent Practice*. Boston, MA: Allyn and Bacon, pp. 225–68.

Hernández, P., Almeida, R., and Vecchio, D. D. (2005) Critical consciousness, accountability, and empowerment: Key processes for helping families heal. *Family Process*, 44 (1): 105–19.

Hill Collins, P. (2000) *Black Feminist Thought: Knowledge, Consciousness, and the Politics of Empowerment*. 2nd edn. New York, NY: Routledge.

Jones, C. and Shorter-Gooden, K. (2003) Shifting: *The Double Lives of Black Women in America*. New York: Harper Collins.

Lewis, C. and Truelar, H. (2008) Rethinking the role of African American churches as social service providers. *Black Theology*, 6: 343–65.

Lykes, M. B. and Moane, G. (2009) Editors' introduction: Whither feminist liberation psychology? Critical explorations of feminist and liberation psychologies for a globalizing world. *Feminism and Psychology*, 19 (3): 283–98.

Martín-Baró, I. (1994) Towards a Liberation Psychology. In A. Aron and S. Corne (eds). *Writings for a Liberation Psychology: Ignacio Martín-Baró*. Cambridge, MA: Harvard University Press, pp. 17–32.

Martín-Baró, I. (1996) *Writings for a Liberation Psychology*. Trans. S. Corne and A. Aron. Cambridge, MA: Harvard Univ. Press.

Mattis, J. S. (2002) Religion and spirituality in the meaning making and coping experiences of African American women: A qualitative analysis. *Psychology of Women Quarterly*, 26: 308–20.

Mbiti, J. S. (1990) *African Religions and Philosophy*. London: Heinemann Educational.

Moane, G. (2003) Bridging the personal and the political: Practices for a liberation psychology. *American Journal of Community Psychology*, 31 (1–2): 91–101.

Moane, G. (2011) *Gender and Colonialism: A Psychological Analysis of Oppression and Liberation*. 2nd edn. Basingstoke: Palgrave/Macmillan.

Montero, M. (1990) Ideology and psychological research in Third World contexts. *Journal of Social Issues*, 36: 43–55.

Murphy, P. (2009) Texas Public School Counselors' Perceptions of Family Strengths in African American Hurricane Katrina Evacuee Children and Adolescents: A Qualitative Study. (Unpublished doctoral dissertation). Denton, TX: Texas Woman's University.

Nobles, W. (1986) *African Psychology: Toward its Reclamation, Reascension and Revitalization*. Princeton, NJ: Institute for Advanced Study.

Parham, T. A. (2002) *Counseling Persons of African Descent: Raising the Bar of Practitioner Competence*. Thousand Oaks, CA: Sage.

Pew Forum (2009) A religious portrait of African Americans. *Religion and Public Life Project*, January 30. Available online at http://pewforum.org/docs/?DocID=389 (accessed October 4, 2013).

Starks, S. and Hughey, A. (2003) African American women at midlife: The relationship between spirituality and life satisfaction. *Affilia*, 18 (2): 133–47.

Taylor, R., Chatters, L. M., and Levin, J. S. (2004) *Religion in the Lives of African Americans: Social, Psychological, and Health Perspectives.* Thousand Oaks, CA: Sage.

US Bureau of the Census. (2011) *Current Population Survey, Annual Social and Economic Supplement, 2010* [Data File]. Available online at www2.census.gov/census_2010. Retrieved January 8, 2012, from http://quickfacts.census.gov./datasets/ Summary_File_1/ 0Final_National/

8

WORKING WITH UPPER-MIDDLE AND PRIVILEGED-CLASS FAMILIES

Eleana McMurry

Introduction to the population: upper-middle-class families

Laszloffy (2008) writes that "class is like the air we breathe" (p. 51). Yet today, in a society in which class lines are blurred by ever-widening income gaps and a culture of consumerism that spans class lines, it is increasingly hard to define usefully ubiquitous terms such as "middle class," "working class," or even "wealthy" (hooks 2000; Laszloffy 2008). Although class differences, as well as economic inequality and segregation, have become more pronounced in the United States, many Americans still believe that we live in a classless society and that economic (upward) mobility is possible for all (hooks 2000). The use of terms such as the "99 percent" or the "1 percent," while they reflect heightened economic disparities and promote solidarity, also blur class definitions (Lichtenstein 2012). Many Americans describe themselves as middle class, despite widely varying definitions of what constitutes this commonly used term.

Class can be measured by several main factors, including income, accrued wealth, education, and occupation; it is not as simple as household income (Laszloffy 2008; Scott and Leonhardt 2005). Today, more than ever, intangibles such as educational opportunities, social education, and social capital matter in predicting and defining class (Scott and Leonhardt 2005). For the purposes of this chapter, "middle class" will be loosely defined as families with household incomes between US$38,000 and US$60,000 per year; upper-middle-class, between US$60,000 and US$100,000; and upper class, between US$100,000 and US$250,000 per year (Levine 2012). Ultra-wealthy members of the upper class, termed "privileged class" in this chapter, refer to families with household incomes over US$250,000 per year.

This chapter looks at upper-middle and privileged-class families from a liberation health perspective. Such individuals and families are, by their very definition, those who benefit the most from the current social, political and economic status quo in America. However, they are not immune to personal, cultural, and institutional pressures that are a result of living in a capitalistic consumer driven society. Upper-middle and privileged-class individuals value and are at the mercy of a culture of hyper-consumerism, professionalism, competition, and individualism. Money and economic privilege do not guarantee happiness. In fact, upper-middle and privileged-class individuals are no more likely to be happy than their working-class or middle-class counterparts (Buss 2000). Materialism alters our human relationships and our capacity to connect as human beings (hooks 2000; Luthar 2003). Upper-middle and privileged-class individuals are susceptible to feelings of isolation, depression, anxiety, eating disorders, and substance abuse, among others (Luthar 2003; Wolfe and Fodor 1996).

The following case study, formulation and literature review provide insight into the personal, cultural and institutional forces that impact the lives and mental health challenges faced by upper-middle and privileged-class families and individuals. The liberation health model is particularly useful in understanding the ways that dominant worldview messaging reinforces the coveted power and privilege afforded upper-middle and privileged-class communities, while at the same time acting as a negative force in the mental health and quality of life of these same communities.

Literature review

This literature review explores the ways in which the very attributes that upper-middle and privileged-class individuals often aspire to simultaneously foster their material success while also having etiological implications for various mental health challenges.

Individualism and isolation

American culture is deeply rooted in the Anglo-American ideal of rugged individualism, the notion that there is opportunity for everyone and that no matter what class we originate in, we can be upwardly mobile (hooks 2000; McGill and Pearce 1996). With its origins in historically Anglo-American power structures and values, individualism remains particularly strong amongst upper-middle and privileged-class Anglo-Americans families; it is today one of the dominant cultural features in American society (McGill and Pearce 1996). This exaggerated "hyper-individualism" drives a culture in which individuals are measured by their achievements and their ability to be self-reliant and financially independent (Luthar 2003; McGill and Pearce 1996: 451). Individual accomplishments are prized and encouraged at a young age (hooks 2000; Luthar 2003). Children in upper-middle-class communities often participate in multiple extracurricular activities with the hope of being well-rounded and successful individuals (Luthar 2003; Luthar, Shoum and Brown 2006). Upper-middle and privileged-class children and adolescents are encouraged to participate in dance, clubs, sports, arts, even volunteerism, as avenues to cultivate achievements and as indicators of future individual success (Luthar 2003). As adults, the culture of hyper-individualism allows such individuals to see themselves as products of their own hard work, not of their privilege (hooks 2000; Laszloffy 2008; McIntosh 2009).

While hyper-individualism breeds self-reliance and self-containment, these qualities present real barriers to coping with failure and deficits. For upper-middle and privileged-class families, problems within the family unit are viewed in the context of the individual and not of the whole unit; individuals are expected to fix their own problems (McGill and Pearce 1996). Failures are felt and experienced individually, not communally (Waldegrave 1998). In upper-middle and privileged-class communities, families and individuals place a premium on maintaining the appearance that they do not have problems. The culture of individualism dictates that personal success is uniquely and wholly a product of one's own efforts, but this belief system also dictates that failures of any kind are the result of personal failing (McGill and Pearce 1996). When individual achievement is a measure of self-worth, upper-middle and privileged-class individuals can interpret failures and disappointment as evidence that they themselves are a failure as a person (Luthar 2003). Exaggerated self-blame, in conjunction with an emphasis on privacy and a preoccupation with one's presentation to the outside world, can leave individuals with heightened feelings of shame, isolation, stress and depression (Brown 2007).

The impact of the culture of hyper-individualism is especially important to consider in working with upper-middle and privileged-class women. Simultaneously encouraged to pursue unprecedented individual achievements in the workforce and also to be perfect and blissful mothers, upper-middle and privileged-class women attempt to excel in multiple arenas (Cain 2009; Everingham, Stevenson, and Warner-Smith 2007; Luthar 2003; Ussher 2010). Girls and young women are increasingly encouraged to ambitiously pursue successful careers and to internalize the promise that they can do and be anything they want. However, women participating as workers in a male dominated capitalist economy continue to experience gender discrimination in most fields, especially in the upper echelons of management (Chonody and Siebert 2008). Despite this reality, upper-middle and privileged-class women who internalize a culture of individualism are prone to assign disproportionate self-blame in the face of unachieved goals. The mental health consequences of these realities are numerous: increased stress and anxiety, substance abuse, depression, and shame (McGill and Pearce 1996; Ussher 2010).

"Keeping up with the Joneses" – competition and perfectionism

Martín-Baró (1994) explains that the needs of a social class are developed through an inherently political socialization process. This socialization reinforces the political and social status quo. It also reinforces the cultural norms and values that are often magnified in upper-middle and privileged-class families. Lives that revolve around individual achievements foster a culture of competition (Luthar 2003). A deeply entrenched socialization of competition and consumerism are woven throughout American life, fostering efforts to "keep up" through the acquisition of prescribed achievement and the participation in patterns of consumption related to clothing, electronics, cars, vacations, homes and the like.

Upper-middle and privileged-class families, like many Americans, tend to compare themselves to those who have more, believing that having more will lead to greater happiness (Csikszentmihalyi 1999). Despite evidence that suggests otherwise, there is a core belief that ownership of goods and acquisition of wealth are essential for happiness (Csikszentmihalyi 1999; Goldbart, Jaffe and DiFuria 2004; Luthar 2003). For children in upper-middle and privileged-class families, a culture of competition and conformity is modeled, encouraged, and replicated later in life (McGill and Pearce 1996). Men in particular are encouraged to be significantly work driven. Despite the rise in dual-income households, and women's increased presence in the workforce, men continue to be expected to be the primary breadwinners (Luthar and Latendresse 2005; McGill and Pearce 1996). Dominant worldview messaging for these men dictates longer hours at the office, excessively competitive work environments, and difficulty in saying no to work opportunities that offer increase in pay or status. Though the drive to attain wealth and status reflects an intense competitiveness and belief that more is better, fear of loss is also a primary motivator: loss of wealth, loss of status, loss of employment, and loss of identity (Golbart, *et al.* 2004; Luthar 2003; McGill and Pearce 1996). Despite relative security, upper-middle and privileged-class individuals can entertain persuasive fears surrounding the prospect of losing money or status (Golbart, *et al.* 2004).

For women, the culture of competition as well as achievement-derived identities, inculcate an "excessive perfectionism" (Luthar and Becker 2002: 1595). For upper-middle and privileged-class women, the desire to be perfect and to "have it all" can be intense: a successful career, a great body, fashionable clothes and accessories, the fairytale wedding, a perfect marriage, and, of course, perfect children (Clarke 2006; McGoldrick 2008; Stoppard 2010). Women in this population can engage in constant self-improvement projects (Brown 2007; Coontz 1992). Even activities from which one might normally derive pleasure become avenues to self-improvement: reading, book clubs, yoga, exercise, travel, etc. Each benchmark of success, worldliness, or beauty is yet another way to make oneself "marketable" to prospective schools, employers, partners. In this, women come to see themselves and be seen as marketable products. This use of sales and advertising language in the way women present themselves is indicative of the ways in which self-worth is tied to achievement.

This culture of perfectionism is visible in upper-middle and privileged-class mothers who remain and excel in high-pressure, male-dominated careers, while placing unrealistic expectations on themselves to be perfect mothers (Everingham, *et al.* 2007; Luthar 2003). Anxiety, depression, and substance abuse are endemic among upper-middle and privileged-class women (Luthar 2003; Ussher 2010). High risk for eating disorders reflects the intense pressures to be thin and conform to dominant messaging surrounding beauty (Luthar 2003).

Barriers to treatment: The "stiff upper lip," stigma, and individualism

Upper-middle and privileged-class families face several barriers in seeking treatment. In an effort to maintain a "veneer of perfection" or to look as "normal" as possible, individuals and families may use treatment as a last resort, when it is no longer possible to deny a problem or when efforts to manage the problem have failed (Luthar 2003: 1590; McGill and Pearce 1996). This is reflective of a fear that formal acknowledgement of problems may negatively impact the long-term educational and professional goals (Luthar 2003; Luthar and Latendresse 2005; McGill and Pearce 1996). Shame, embarrassment, and fear of gossip all reinforce the stigma created by dominant worldview messaging.

Upper-middle and privileged-class individuals, particularly Anglo-Americans, also believe that individual problems should be dealt with individually. There is a certain amount of pride associated with self-containment, particularly surrounding sharing negative emotions. Sharing one's emotional world can feel distasteful or frightening, even for those voluntarily attending and paying for therapy. Individuals may feel that sharing too much about themselves will burden others: "they would rather not complain" (McGill and Pearce 1996: 452). Maintaining a "stiff upper lip," while perhaps beneficial in professional environments, can serve to isolate families and individuals and reinforce stigma and shame, all in the service of privacy. Conversely, some affluent families and individuals readily utilize mental health services, often in the way of private therapists. Although perhaps not trying to deal with problems on their own, heavy use of individual therapy is also reflective of the feeling that problems arise from individual pathology, rather than society at large. In a sense, paying for individual therapy allows individuals to seek help without having to reach out to friends or community; this act not can not only rob people of an opportunity for more interdependence, but again reinforces the notion that the problem lies within the individual not within the environment.

Finally, upper-middle and privileged-class individuals are aware of the question: What could they possibly be unhappy about? Many, including upper-middle and privileged-class individuals themselves, may place judgment on the problems that they face in a life of relative security and as those who benefit the most from the status quo (Glick 2012; Goldbart, et al. 2004). Additionally, clinicians are more likely to minimize or dismiss symptoms of upper-middle and privileged-class individuals (Luthar 2003; Luthar and Latendresse 2005; Pollak and Shafer 1985). Individuals seeking treatment are likely to be aware of unsympathetic societal views of them: That they have no one to blame but themselves, that they are entitled, arrogant, selfish, superficial (Goldbart, et al. 2004; Luthar 2003). These stereotypes follow individuals to treatment and can serve to minimize very real problems (Luthar 2003; Luthar and Latendresse 2005).

Case presentation

Introduction to the context

Nancy is a 53-year-old married, heterosexual, white woman living in a wealthy suburb of a major urban center on the East coast. Nancy lives with her husband and has been diagnosed with major depressive disorder. Nancy has two children, both of whom are college age.

Referral and presenting problem

Nancy was referred for outpatient mental health services immediately following a seven-day admission to an inpatient psychiatric treatment unit. Nancy was admitted for worsening depression and passive suicidal ideation. The admission was the culmination of worsening anxiety and depression over the past year and a half that left both her husband and her primary-care physician concerned for her welfare.

I first met Nancy during her intake at the outpatient mental health center, following her seven-day inpatient psychiatric unit stay. For the past seven months, Nancy has continued outpatient treatment on a weekly basis. The following case presentation reflects Nancy's story following these seven months of outpatient treatment.

Current situation

Both Nancy's husband and primary-care physician prompted Nancy's most recent admission to the psychiatric treatment unit and referral to outpatient mental health services; both had become increasingly concerned by Nancy's experience of depression. During the initial assessment in the outpatient center, Nancy stated that she felt her depression was worsening and was preventing her from facing many of her daily tasks. Nancy stated that initially she enjoyed herself after her youngest child left for college. She had joined a book club in her community and had begun making travel plans for the future. Nancy recounted that overall, she felt energetic and excited about this next chapter in her life. Four months later, Nancy felt increasingly lethargic. Her thoughts turned to negative self-talk. She began to feel that she "did not want to be here."

While Nancy had had episodes of depression in the past, she indicated that her experience of her depression was amplified after her children left home. In our ongoing discussions about what had generated the symptoms of depression, Nancy stated that the depression had "snuck up on her." During our sessions, Nancy was able to identify a marked increase in symptoms following her children's return to school after winter break. She recalled noting that the depression was "really getting bad" at the point that she could not get out of bed or perform the most simple of tasks. She also noted that her husband had recently taken on increased responsibilities at work, which meant more income for the household, but also less time together at home. As we continued to discuss her experience of depression, Nancy noted that when her children lived at home, she felt she had more of a purpose. Further, she was better able to manage her depression because she was busy all the time. Without that structure that her children's schedules provided, Nancy acknowledged that she felt lost, "blue," and unmotivated to do things that brought her enjoyment.

Nancy expressed her feelings of embarrassment and bewilderment over her recent struggles with depression. She wondered why she could not just "hold it together." During family meetings, her husband and Mary, their eldest child, conveyed their surprise at her recent struggles. Her husband knew she had struggled with depression in the past, but her children "had no idea." Both her husband and daughter agreed that on the outside Nancy looked happy. Nancy had been seeing a therapist in recent years, initially to help her through "some difficult years of adolescence" experienced by her son who had abused substances in high school. Nancy noted that she stopped going to counseling when things got better with her son. As we further explored her feelings of depression and hopelessness, Nancy expressed discomfort with her life and stated that she felt that she had no purpose.

Individual and family history

Nancy grew up in a middle-class suburban neighborhood in the same metropolitan area she lives in today. Until the time of her birth, Nancy's mother was a school-teacher; her father was an auto parts salesman. While she describes her childhood as a happy one, she also acknowledges that her father struggled with depression and drank heavily, often stumbling to bed. There were occasional arguments in the home, usually related to her father's drinking. Nancy grew up in a homogeneous (white) neighborhood, which she describes as relatively boring but "safe." Nancy was a very social child and recalls spending a lot of time playing at the homes of other children, often to avoid the tension in her own home. During high school, Nancy was very active in school. Both of her parents were college graduates and had high expectations for their only child. Nancy met this challenge with a perfect grade-point average and acceptance to a regional women's liberal arts school. Nancy identified her senior year in high school as the time when she first started to feel symptoms of depression, stating that she was "overwhelmed by daily tasks" and feelings of unworthiness.

When Nancy was in college, her mother began to work as a teacher part time. Though it was never said explicitly, Nancy believed that this was a way for her mother to "escape" her father at home. Nancy graduated at the top of her class in college, but remained undecided as to her future career. She dated a few men while in college, but "no one she fancied." She moved back in with her parents after college. Nancy described the year that followed as her first major episode of depression. She tutored some of her mother's students part-time for spending money, and came to hate living at home. She became isolative and "exhausted." This is when she first went to see a psychiatrist, though she characterized this interaction as "not helpful." Early in our sessions, Nancy recalled "just snapping out of it one day." In her narrative, she "pulled [her]self up" and began the process of applying to law school. At a time when law schools were actively recruiting women, she soon found herself with a scholarship and new sense of accomplishment and assurance. Her depression dissipated.

In law school, Nancy met Frank. They were married shortly after graduation. Both Nancy and Frank worked after passing the bar: Nancy in a government position, Frank at a law firm. Nancy worked part-time after the birth of her first child, a daughter. After the birth of her second child, a son, Nancy left her work and devoted herself to motherhood. She indicated that she felt that being a stay-at home mother was what was expected of her, but also felt conflicted as a woman with an advanced degree "wasting her talents." As a young mother, Nancy recalled feeling lonely, depressed and isolated at times, but experienced her depression as manageable. While Nancy was at home with her children, Frank continued to work long hours at the same law firm, eventually affording them financial security and a home in an upper-middle-class suburb. Nancy and Frank were able to send their children to private high schools and enroll them in many extracurricular activities. Nancy described her children's lives, and by extension, her life, as extremely busy and filled with soccer games, tennis lessons, ballet practice, etc. In our conversations together, Nancy reflected that her busyness allowed her to push her feelings of depression away. Despite some difficulties during her children's teen years, particularly substance use by her son, Nancy stated that being a mother made her feel "worthwhile." A few months after her youngest child went to college, Nancy began to experience increased symptoms of depression. While she initially tried to busy herself through her book club and by future travel plans, eventually her depression became unmanageable, ultimately culminating in her in-patient admission.

Formulation

Nancy's experience of depression is primarily characterized by feelings of unworthiness, purposelessness, general sense of lethargy, and a tendency to isolate and push aside self-care needs. Nancy is engaged in outpatient treatment due to her recognition that her depression has become unmanageable and overwhelming. Nancy's story is that she alone is responsible for her depression. However, a confluence of personal, cultural and institutional factors contribute to her worsening feelings of depression.

Nancy's feelings of depression are influenced by a number of personal factors. She likely has some significant genetic loading for depression. In addition to this predisposition to depression, other personal factors, both past and present, are also powerful contributors. Nancy's recent loss of her role as a full-time mother and caretaker, her life as the partner of a workaholic, her feelings of disconnection from her family, and her concerns about her youngest child are all contributors.

Personal Factors

- Adult Child of an alcoholic
- Genetic loading for depression
- Children recently moved out of the home
- Husband is a workaholic/ works too much
- Loss and grief related to loss of role as a mother

- Physical and psychological symptoms of depression
- Feeling disconnected from husband and children

Cultural Factors

- Gender roles: mother in a hetero-normative family, wife, caretaker
- Culture of perfectionism: Notion that women should "have it all"
- Stigma surrounding depression and alcoholism
- "Keeping up with the Jones"
- Culture of consumerism
- Culture of individualism
- Myth of meritocracy

Institutional Factors

- Capitalism
- Institution of marriage
- For-profit health care system

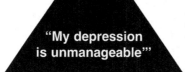

"My depression is unmanageable'"

FIGURE 8.1 Working with upper–middle and privileged class families
Source: Eleana McMurry

Furthermore, Nancy's childhood in an alcoholic home continues to impact her life and feelings about herself in the present. Nancy indicates that she has never fully dealt with how her father's alcoholism impacted her world view and sense of self.

Nancy's youngest child recently went away to college, leaving Nancy with a profound sense of loss. Having been a full-time caretaker for the past 18 years, Nancy is in many ways mourning the loss of her role as a mother, feeling that she hadn't really "thought it through" and "does not know what to do" with herself. The loss of her full time job as a caretaker reawakens the feelings of regret she has over giving up her career many years ago. Nancy's sense of loss and regret is exacerbated also by her husband's work schedule. His increased responsibilities at his law firm translate into even longer hours at the office and more solitude for Nancy. Nancy is increasingly isolated in her wealthy suburb from both family and community. Furthermore, Nancy reports being "fraught with worry" about her youngest child who was suspended for drinking at school during his senior year of high school. Although he is in college now, Nancy continues to worry that her son will develop an alcohol problem like her father; this worry creates feelings of powerlessness and helplessness in Nancy similar to those she felt as a young person.

In addition to the personal factors contributing to Nancy's depression, there are powerful cultural forces at work in Nancy's life. Gender roles, stigma and shame surrounding her own depression and her father's alcoholism, a culture of perfectionism, the isolation of suburban life, and a constant pressure to "keep up with the Joneses" all weigh heavily on Nancy. Cultural messaging surrounding gender roles and what it means to be a woman and a mother seep into every facet of Nancy's life and understanding of herself. As a young person, Nancy felt pressure to be a perfect daughter: accomplished educationally, beautiful, and obedient to her parents, and she succeeded. She succeeded subsequently as a professional and as a suburban mother. What is she succeeding at now?

As an adult, Nancy struggles with cultural messaging about what it means to be a good mother, a good wife and an accomplished woman. Nancy cites feelings of inadequacy when she thinks about a need to be "the whole package" and "put together." Nancy reflects that in her community pressure to maintain a certain body image and projection of wealth are "exhausting to keep up with," especially as she ages. Nancy not only feels pressure to feel perfect herself, but also admits to struggling with the feeling that her children, as reflections of herself, need to be perfect. Conflicting cultural messaging about the roles of women and mothers, as well as the pressure to fit in in her wealthy suburban community, not only leave little room for authenticity or individuality, but also leave Nancy feeling depressed and inadequate.

While Nancy feels the pressures of looking and playing the part of a perfect wife and mother, she also feels significant shame and regret about giving up her career as an attorney, feeling at times that her life as lawyer might have been more meaningful. Cultural value placed on productivity weighs heavily on Nancy and is a source of negative feelings about herself. Nancy acknowledges that she sometimes blames herself for not being "superwoman," pursuing both motherhood and her legal career. Perhaps most damaging to Nancy is her belief that she must deal with her depression on her own and put on a good face for the outside world. A culture of individualism and self-sufficiency disempowers Nancy as an agent of change in her own life. Immersed in dominant cultural messages, Nancy is reluctant to seek help or solidarity in her community, choosing instead to conceal her struggles with depression.

There are also significant institutional factors contributing to Nancy's feelings of depression and inadequacy. While she and her family have materially benefited from educational and legal institutions, Nancy has complicated relationships with the institutions of marriage and capitalism. Her role as a mother and the feelings of loss she now experiences as an "empty nester" are inextricably bound to the institution of the tightly bounded nuclear family. Similarly, life in a capitalistic system privileges her as an upper-class individual, but it also creates distance and competition amongst would-be friends and feelings of inadequacy regarding her choice to give up a lucrative law career to care for her children.

Frank's long hours and drive to "provide the very best" for his family ultimately means he is not present as a partner much of the time. Nancy's and Frank's socioeconomic status shores up a marriage that increasingly feels to Nancy like a financial and gendered division of labor arrangement. Further, modern-day capitalism devalues Nancy as a mother, and also drives a family life in which her husband is rewarded for being a workaholic. Both Nancy and her husband feel the pressure of upward mobility, measuring themselves through their accumulation of capital (security) and consumer products. Though Nancy and her family continue to thrive economically in a capitalist system, she nonetheless experiences feelings of inadequacy and depression that are driven by consumerism and the institutional underpinnings of capitalism and heteronormative marriage.

The convergence of the personal, cultural and institutional factors in Nancy's life not only contribute to her feelings of depression but also deeply impact the way she makes sense of her life.

Interventions

Consciousness-raising: Broadening of the issue beyond the personal and individual

During our time together, Nancy and I discussed barriers to her treatment and the need to challenge her beliefs about depression. We focused on three main ways that dominant worldview messaging impacted her depression: a culture of individualism, gender roles and cultures of perfectionism and competition.

Initially, I asked Nancy how she had tried to manage her depression on her own. I also asked her why she delayed asking for help, both at first onset of symptoms and once she began experiencing more severe feelings of depression. Initially Nancy responded with "I don't know" and "I felt like it was my problem and I should handle it." In further discussions, Nancy conceded that she was raised to "always rely on myself because when the chips are down, all you have is yourself." Moreover, Nancy felt that she did not have anyone close to her that she felt comfortable talking to about it.

Deconstructing the culture of individualism with Nancy, we discussed the ways in which the value of self-reliance is instilled in many of us at an early age. We discussed the ways in which internalized messages about individualism and self-reliance benefited her and the ways in which it made it difficult for her to reach out for help. Nancy identified a number of areas where a culture of individualism was pervasive in her life. Nancy saw the ways in which individualism drove her towards personal achievements and the ways in which it undermined some of her emotional needs. Looking back, notions of self-reliance prevented her both from seeking much needed help at a time of personal crisis, and from getting timely help for her son when he was struggling with substance use in high school. Nancy shared that she was raised with a "pull yourself up by your bootstraps" approach to life and conceded that she felt "like such a burden" at home after her hospitalization. While she felt profoundly lonely prior the hospitalization, she now felt uncomfortable with the attention paid to her by her children and husband.

Deconstructing dominant worldview messaging around gender roles was also important in addressing aspects of Nancy's experience with depression. During intake, Nancy had identified difficulties she experienced as a mother and acknowledged occasional ambivalence towards her decision to be a homemaker. Nancy was reluctant to express aspects of mothering that were difficult for her. When I initially asked Nancy whether she felt that gender roles might have impacted her struggles with depression, she rushed to assure me that she really loves being a mother and that she was grateful that she could be fully involved as her children grow up. At this point, Nancy was completely comfortable in acknowledging the loneliness that was created as a result of feeling the need to "fix [herself]," but uncomfortable with critiquing any aspect of her roles as a mother. Nancy and I discussed messaging about women who are ambivalent about mothering, namely that they "are bad mothers." I added: "Because all mothers should be saints and love every second of being a mother, right?" Nancy laughed and conceded that she had not loved every minute.

During another session, Nancy and I discussed the ways in which her day-to-day life reflected normative gender roles. After her children went away to school, she found herself thinking about her relationship with her husband. She had begun to resent the fact that he worked so much. Nancy could think of lots of reasons her husband should keep working: college tuition bills, adding to a retirement fund. However, Nancy was also lonely at home.

In further discussions, Nancy reflected on the reality that it would have never occurred to her and her husband to discuss the possibility of his staying at home when their children were born. They both had assumed that she would be the one to scale back her employment. I asked: "In whose interest is it for women to be full time caretakers? Who benefits when mothers hold themselves to the unattainable expectation of 'supermom'?" Nancy, coming to life with some humorous anecdotes, recounted the ways in which caretaking roles automatically fell to women. While Nancy found humor in her own life as a caretaker, she also acknowledged that these roles had decreased her earning power and her financial independence. Although Nancy was concerned mainly with the loss of earning power as a result of giving up her legal career, it is worth noting that, as a homemaker and full-time mother, Nancy did in fact engage in full-time work, albeit unpaid and unrecognized as contributing to the economic system, one which is supported and sustained by the unpaid and undervalued labor of women.

Nancy was able to identify stressors that she faced as a result of cultural messaging about gender, particularly those related to motherhood and her assumed role as the caretaker of her husband and children. She could see how these stressors had negatively impacted her self-esteem and mental health: increased workload in the home, increased social isolation, and high expectations surrounding being a wife and mother.

Finally, I asked Nancy whether she felt perfectionism and competition affected her depression. Nancy and I discussed the ways in which dominant messaging drove her need to "act the part" – to look a certain way, to dress a certain way, to drive a certain car, for children to have certain possessions, to live in a certain neighborhood. Nancy communicated that she found conspicuous consumption distasteful, but she and her husband had been "worn down" over the years by the pressure to "keep up with the Joneses," particularly as it related to their children. The atmosphere at her children's school was such that consumption and accumulation of "stuff" just seemed to be the norm; many of her purchases were driven by what "the other kids' parents were doing." We discussed the ways in which consumer culture shapes our perceived needs. I asked her whether she felt that these pressures had a positive or a negative impact on her depression. Would she feel relief if no longer felt that she had to keep up with the Joneses? Nancy felt that external pressures of any kind were "not great" for her depression. She felt that the longer her children were in college, the more opportunity she would have to work on shedding some of the external pressures of "keeping up."

Now, spending a great deal of time alone, Nancy worried that she did not meet her full potential as a lawyer. I asked Nancy why she felt she should do it all. Why was this the ideal life? Nancy felt that there was a sense that women can and should do it all. Nancy conceded while she missed the actual work, she also missed the prestigious identity she garnered as a lawyer. We discussed grief as a natural reaction to giving up a career. We then talked about the idea of "superwoman," who has and does it all. Nancy ultimately decided that no one can really have and do it all.

Developing community

One of the most transformative aspects of Nancy's looking at the beliefs she held about herself is that she began to see her problems as ones that affected not only her, but many women. Nancy and I spoke about ways in which she could feel a part of the community at large that did not involve her children. Nancy had already started attending a book club, and while she found it intimidating in some ways she was excited by the opportunity to be intellectually stimulated and to have conversations that did not revolve around her family life.

Nancy and I explored this desire for community and solidarity further. I suggested a support group for women with depression or some kind of work, volunteer or otherwise that might connect Nancy to other like-minded women. Nancy was initially averse to a support group, afraid she might see someone she knows, but eventually considered going to one in a nearby town. Nancy was much more excited by the idea of working. Although she would not be able to practice law, Nancy began to brainstorm ways she could use her legal expertise in some kind of volunteer capacity. Nancy reached out to acquaintances who had had legal careers in the public sector to ask about volunteer ideas. A number of possibilities presented themselves, including work through a local charity providing legal aid to refugees and immigrants applying for residency, asylum, or citizenship. She committed to beginning as a volunteer as soon as possible. Engaging in these types of activities served a two-fold purpose for Nancy: she was able to begin to forge a new identity through new activities, while also allowing herself the chance to create community and support for herself.

Taking action

While one of the primary ways in which Nancy took action was seeking out opportunities in the community and creating a sense of belonging and purpose for herself outside of the home, there were also dynamics in her personal relationships that no longer worked for her. Coping with the loss of a career in the wake of the loss of her role as a full-time caretaker was very important for Nancy. While taking steps to find new roles for herself in the community was one step, Nancy had made clear that she also needed to renegotiate her relationship with her family, specifically her husband. Traditional roles, found in the hetero-normative nuclear family in which the male "provides" and the woman caretakes, no longer served them as a couple. While it was clear that in many ways these roles did not ever serve Nancy well, Nancy and Frank were now both faced with a stasis in which neither of their roles fit their current life: they did not need Frank to work full time and they no longer had children in the house for whom Nancy provided care.

During the time that we worked together, Nancy did not undertake a conversation about renegotiating roles with her husband, from whom she felt increasingly distant. While I could see value in renegotiating aspects of their relationship, for reasons I can only surmise, Nancy was not ready or not interested in broaching this at the time. It can be said that for anyone, letting go of long-standing ways of relating and living is a process that does not happen overnight. In the case of Nancy, she may have ambivalence about asking her husband to let go of perceived power, money and prestige; she herself may have ambivalence about decisions that impact their relative financial security and comfort. Moreover, it is possible that she does not see any possibility for change in their marriage.

Personal reflection

I have always found the liberation health model to be a natural fit when addressing the problems of individuals who are members of marginalized populations. It is a compelling, social justice-oriented, and inclusive model that reflects the lived realities of our clients: the realities not taken into consideration in the diagnostic-driven healthcare model so prevalent today. Initially, I worried that this model seemed less obvious or relevant in its possible application to the problems of those we think of as actually benefiting from the current status quo: upper-middle-class and privileged-class individuals. In reflecting on Nancy's struggles and my own upper-middle-class upbringing, I once again grappled with my class privilege and was struck that dominant messaging still filters so much of what I do, think, and take in. As a part of this process, I reflected on how the culture of individualism, competition, and consumerism influence my thinking and even my own feelings about my work. I love and am committed to social work as a profession and a way of being in the world; yet I still second-guess my decision to do this work, because a voice tells me that I should have gone into a more lucrative, status-driven career. It is the dominant worldview messaging, churning away in the back of my consciousness and whispering to me that my productivity is intricately tied to my self-worth.

References

Brown, B. (2007) *I Thought it was Just Me (But it Isn't)*. New York: Penguin.

Buss, D. (2000) The evolution of happiness. *American Psychologist*, 55 (1): 15–23.

Cain, R. (2009) "A view you won't get anywhere else?" Depressed mothers, public regulation and 'private' narrative. *Feminist Legal Studies*, 17 (2): 123–43.

Chonody, J. M. and Siebert, D. C. (2008) Gender differences in depression: A theoretical examination of power. *Affilia: Journal of Women and Social Work*, 23 (4): 338–48.

Clarke, H. (2006) Depression: Women's sadness or high-prevalence disorder? *Australian Social Work*, 59 (4): 365–77.

Coontz, S. (1992) The Way We Never Were: American Families and the Nostalgia Trap, 2nd edn. New York: Basic Books.

Csikszentmihalyi, M. (1999) If we are so rich, why aren't we happy? *American Psychologist*, 54 (10): 821–7.

Everingham, C., Stevenson, D., and Warner-Smith, P. (2007) "Things are getting better all the time?" Challenging the narrative of women's progress from a generational perspective. *Sociology*, 41 (3): 419–37.

Glick, R. A. (2012) The rich are different: Issues of wealth in analytic treatments. In B. Berger, and S. Newman (eds), *Money Talks: In Therapy, Society, and Life*. New York: Routledge, pp. 21–33.

Goldbart, S., Jaffe, D. T., and DiFuria, J. (2004) Money, meaning, and identity: Coming to terms with being wealthy. In T. Kasser, and A. D. Kanner (eds) , *Psychology and Consumer Culture: The Struggle For a Good Life in a Materialistic World*. Washington, DC: American Psychological Association, pp. 189–210.

hooks, b. (2000) *Where We Stand: Class Matters*. New York: Routledge.

Laszloffy, T. A. (2008) Social class: Implications for family therapy. In M. McGoldrick (ed.), *Re-visioning Family Therapy*, 2nd edn. New York: Guilford Press, pp. 48–60.

Levine, L. (2012). *The Distribution of Household Income and the Middle Class*. Washington, DC: Congressional Research Service. Available online at http://assets.opencrs.com/rpts/RS20811_20121113.pdf (October 4, 2013).

Lichtenstein, N. (2012) Class unconsciousness: Stop using "middle class" to depict the labor movement. *New Labor Forum*, 21 (2): 10–13.

Luthar, S. S. (2003) The culture of affluence: Psychological costs of material wealth. *Child Development*, 74 (6): 1581–93.

Luthar, S. S., and Becker, B. E. (2002) Privileged but pressured? A study of affluent youth. *Child Development*, 73 (5): 1593–610.

Luthar, S. S., and Latendresse, S. J. (2005) Children of the affluent. *Current Directions in Psychological Science*, 14 (1): 49–53.

Luthar, S. S., Shoum, K. A., and Brown, P. J. (2006) Extracurricular involvement among affluent youth: A scapegoat for "ubiquitous achievement pressures?" *Developmental Psychology*, 42 (3): 583–97.

Martín-Baró, I. (1994) *Writings for a Liberation Psychology*. Cambridge, MA: Harvard University Press.

McGill, D. W. and Pearce, J. K. (1996) American families with English ancestors from the colonial era: Anglo Americans. In M. McGoldrick, J. Giordano and J. Pearce (eds), *Ethnicity and Family Therapy*, 2nd edn. New York: Guilford Press, pp. 427–50.

McGoldrick, M. (2008) Finding a place called "home." In M. McGoldrick (ed.) *Re-visioning Family Therapy*, 2nd edn. New York: Guilford Press, pp. 97–113.

McIntosh, P. (2009) White privilege and male privilege: A personal account of coming to correspondences through work in women. In A. Ferber, C. Jimenez, A. Herrera and D. Samuels (eds) , *The Matrix Reader: Examing the Dynamics of Oppression and Privilege*. New York: McGraw Hill Higher Education, pp. 146–54.

Pollak, J. M. and Schaffer, S. (1985) The mental health clinician in the affluent public school setting. *Clinical Social Work Journal*, 13 (4): 341–55.

Scott, J. and Leonhardt, D. (2005) Shadow lines that still divide. *New York Times*, May 15.

Available online at www.nytimes.com/2005/05/15/national/class/OVERVIEW-FINAL.html?pagewanted=1 (October 4, 2013).

Stoppard, J. M. (2010) I. moving towards an understanding of women's depression. *Feminism and Psychology*, 20 (2): 267–71.

Ussher, J. M. (2010) Are we medicalizing women's misery? A critical review of women's higher rates of reported depression. *Feminism and Psychology*, 20 (1): 9–35.

Waldegrave, C. (1998) The challenges of culture to psychology and postmodern thinking. In M. McGoldrick (ed.), *Re-visioning Family Therapy*, 1st edn. New York: Guilford Press, pp. 405–13.

Wolfe, J. and Fodor, I. G. (1996) The poverty of privilege: Therapy with women of the "upper" classes. *Women and Therapy*, 18 (3/4): 73.

9

LIBERATION HEALTH IN A CHILD PROTECTION AGENCY

Zack Osheroff

Introduction of author and of the institutional context of the case to be presented

This chapter describes the experiences of an intern studying for a master's in social work, Mary, during her time at a public child welfare office, as she tried to address an obstacle to liberation health service delivery. To protect the identities of those involved, Mary's name has been changed and the location has been omitted. Information for the chapter was collected through interviews with Mary. The author, ZJO, holds a masters degree in social work and works with underserved children and families.

Mary's agency is in a rural/suburban area. The agency, a state-level public organization, is tasked with protecting children from abuse and neglect. Not all employees have social work degrees, but many do. After several years as an agency employee, Mary decided to take advantage of an opportunity to earn a master's in social work while interning at her agency. It was in this capacity that Mary decided to take action to positively affect her agency. Over the course of her social work education, Mary came to recognize her responsibility to direct her critical consciousness inwards towards herself and her own agency, and to utilize that information to take action to benefit co-workers and clients. Her story is an illustration of how social workers can work for positive change in the contexts of our own offices and organizations.

Specifically, Mary began to recognize that there was a troubling volume of disrespectful, blaming, and condescending comments made about clients by workers at her agency. The National Association of Social Workers Code of Ethics (NASW 2008) states in Article 1.12, "Social workers should not use derogatory language in their written or verbal communications to or about clients. Social workers should use accurate and respectful language in all communications to and about clients."

While this is the expectation that many people have of social workers, and many social workers have of themselves, living up to it every day presents a challenge and often requires a critical perspective of personal, cultural, and institutional factors and a willingness to act.

Literature review

This review will focus on contextualizing and understanding, from a liberation health perspective, the pervasive negativity about clients that occurred in Mary's agency. We will then be able to consider the steps that Mary took to empower herself and her colleagues to address a dysfunctional aspect of their work. I have organized the literature into three parts: the first is an explanation of the practice of victim blaming that has permeated many social work institutions, and indeed most of mainstream society; the second part examines the concept of burnout in general, and specifically in the child welfare sector; and the last section examines how the particular dynamics of child welfare, such as working with mandated clients and representing state power, effect the social work relationship.

Blaming the victim

When William Ryan wrote *Blaming the Victim* (1971), the conceptualization he created was a new one in sociology, but the practice he identified was very old. Ryan drew attention to an often invisible consequence of dominant worldview messaging and systemic oppression: society's attempt to locate the cause of any particular social problem within those most negatively affected by the problem. Ryan points out that blaming the student of an underperforming urban school for failing to learn is similar to blaming Pearl Harbor for being attacked by the Japanese during World War II; "What was Pearl Harbor doing in the Pacific?" (p. 3).

He illustrates this phenomenon by exploring the social discrimination directed at poor black families, on the apparent assumption that the persistent poverty and inequality they experience are of their own making. This has taken many forms: the caricature of the laziness and conniving of "welfare queens," (Gilliam 1999); the supposedly inherited "culture of poverty," (Gorski 2008); even the biologically based intellectual inferiority of African-descended people (Smedley and Smedley 2005). A landmark example of blaming the victim at the highest levels of society is the 1965 report by Daniel Moynihan on the black family (US Department of Labor, Office of Policy Planning and Research 1965). Specifically, Moynihan states that a family dynamic had developed within the black community as a consequence of its historical and collective experiences of horror under the regimes of chattel slavery and post-reconstruction persecution. This family dynamic was supposedly responsible for the deprivation of opportunities for black folks to lift themselves out of poverty and curb unequal outcomes: "The white family has achieved a high degree of stability and is maintaining that stability. By contrast, the family structure of lower class Negroes is highly unstable, and in many urban centers is approaching complete breakdown" (US Department of Labor, Office of Policy Planning and Research 1965: The Negro American Family section, paras. 1–2, 8–10).

By adopting this narrative, centers of authority were able to obfuscate the active racial prejudice, economic injustice, and social domination visited upon black communities by the dominant culture. This practice continues to this day, with many citizens convinced that equality can be achieved only by "fixing" the oppressed group as opposed to recognizing the real culprits, such as racist institutions, post-industrialization, and the war on drugs. Additionally, members of the dominant culture employ blaming the victim to avoid confronting their own responsibility for, in this instance, perpetuating racism and the social and economic advantages they receive as a consequence.

Popular notions that ultimately blame the impoverished and underserved for the contexts in which they find themselves permeate social work and other service providers in profound ways. Ryan describes an experience he had consulting with volunteers of a program that worked with unwed mothers:

> my first sessions with the staff were taken up with discussions of the strange sexual mores of the lower class black girl, and how to "motivate" clients to get themselves educated, employed, and "off welfare." These kind, sympathetic, and endlessly helpful women were absorbed with the ways in which their clients were different, vulnerable, and problematic, and they were dedicated to helping them adjust to their impossible life circumstances rather than changing the circumstances. They were, in a word, Blaming the Victim.
>
> (Ryan 1971: 87–8)

Despite Ryan's work, blaming the victim has persisted through many notional ideas about the oppressed, such as the "culture of poverty" idea (ibid: 114–18), and can be seen in contemporary academia and mainstream politics (Cohen 2010), as well as among child welfare workers and child protection workers (Derezotes, Poertner, and Testa 2005; Elliott and Urquiza 2006; Johnson and Sullivan 2008).

Burnout

Burnout has received considerable attention in the academic literature for its negative consequences for service delivery and job performance both within and outside the social work profession (Maslach and Jackson 1981; Leiter and Maslach 1988; Shirom 1989; Schaufeli, Bakker and Rhenen 2009; Toppinen-Tanner, Ojajarvi, Vaanaanen, Kalimo, and Jappinen 2005). The term was coined by Freudenberger in 1974, but it was the work of Maslach and others that developed the construct of burnout as it is understood today (Maslach 1982; Maslach and Jackson 1981; Maslach and Pines 1977). Maslach and others considered burnout to be characterized by three interrelated conditions experienced by the worker:

emotional exhaustion, diminished personal accomplishment, and, most relevantly, depersonalization.

Depersonalization is a dehumanizing attitude that workers direct at clients whereby workers treat clients as objects (Cordes and Dougherty 2008; Jackson, Turner, and Brief 1987). It can also be thought of as "the development of negative, cynical attitudes and feelings about one's clients," and can "lead staff to view their clients as somehow deserving of their troubles" (Maslach and Jackson 1981: 99). This is thought to occur as a coping strategy for managing stress by creating distance and detachment (Carver, Scheier, and Weintraub 1989; Roth and Cohen 1986). A primary feature of depersonalization is making negative comments about clients.

Causes of burnout

Many antecedents to burnout have been examined in the literature. Perhaps unsurprisingly, investigation of burnout began with researchers looking to preexisting attributes of workers to understand the origins of burnout. Characteristics, like sex and/or gender, of the individuals experiencing burnout have been studied at length (Maslach and Jackson 1981, 1985; Pretty 1992; Greenglass, Burke, and Ondrach 1990; Norvell, Hills, and Murrin 1993; Hiscott and Connop 1989), age (Maslach and Jackson 1981; Stevens and O'Neill 1983; Zabel and Zabel 1982; Anderson and Iwanicki 1984), and even more abstract personality characteristics such as "neuroticism," low extraversion, agreeableness, conscientiousness, and openness have been examined (Maslach, Schaufeli, and Leiter 2001; Piedmont 1993; Zellars, Perrewé, and Hochwarter 2000). Other research suggests that workers put themselves at risk of burnout when they do not have realistic expectations for change in their clients (Lamb 1979) or when workers get too "emotionally and psychically involved" with clients (Emener 1979). Even low self-control has been identified as a potential factor leading to burnout (Diestel and Schmidt 2010).

As Arches (1997) points out, however, much of this research and conjecture could be considered to be blaming the victim (in this case, the worker) in its own right, as there is mounting evidence that agencies are, to a large degree, responsible for burnout in their employees. For instance, Arches makes the case that the increasing bureaucratization of service delivery is the culprit. A review of the literature suggests a number of ways that organizations contribute to burnout in their workers.

Many organizational factors have been found to correlate with increased burnout in employees, more than can be enumerated here. Some key findings, however, are particularly pertinent to child welfare workers. For instance, it has been repeatedly found that high role conflict (supervisors communicating incongruous or incompatible expectations to employees), role ambiguity (employees lacking clear communication on proper procedures or evaluation criteria), and role overload (employees feeling that they have neither the time nor skills to meet supervisors' expectations) lead to burnout (Söderfeldt, Söderfeldt, and Warg 1995;

Hansung and Stoner 2008; Schwab and Iwanicki 1982; Maslach and Pines 1977; Russell, Altmaier, and Van Velzen 1987). Additionally, it has been found that issues of autonomy, such as perceptions of lack of control on the job (Glass and Mcknight 1996) and lack of involvement in decision making (Posig and Kickul 2003) are associated with burnout. Workers who feel that they get little positive feedback and gratitude in return for their hard work are more likely to burn out (VanYperen, Buunk, and Schaufeli 1992). Finally, a lack of solidarity among workers and between workers and their organization, such that workers feel alone in being responsible for the future well-being of clients, leads to burnout (Maslach 1982).

Resources that prevent burnout

There are also some important organizational factors that may counteract burnout. These include social support, both formal and informal (Houkes, Janssen, de Jonge, and Bakker 2003), positive supervisor contact (Leiter and Maslach 1988), high-quality supervisor relationship (Bakker, Demerouti, and Euwema 2005), constructive performance feedback (ibid.), worker autonomy (ibid.), and perceived organizational support (Lizano and Barak 2012). It should also be noted that Demerouti, Bakker, Nachreiner, and Schaufeli (2001) considered many factors to be negatively associated specifically with depersonalization. Performance feedback (Åström, Nilsson, Norgerg, and Winblad 1990), rewards (Landsbergis 1988), participation in decision making (Jackson, et al. 1987), and supervisor support (Leiter 1989), in particular, may reduce negative ideas and comments about clients among social workers.

Burnout and public child welfare workers

Public child welfare workers are at increased risk for burnout compared to other social workers (Anderson 2000; Boyas and Wind 2010; McGee 1989; Azar 2000; Stevens and Higgins 2002). In fact, the number of current child welfare workers experiencing compassion fatigue or burnout could be as high as 50 percent (Conrad and Keller-Guenther 2006). Researchers have begun to explore why this might be. Kim (2011) found that public child welfare workers experienced higher workloads, greater role conflict, and had lower personal accomplishment than other social workers. Kim also discovered that public child welfare workers had higher levels of depersonalization than private child welfare workers. According to a study by the US General Accounting Office (2003), public child welfare workers are underpaid, have heavier workloads, poorer working environments, and less adequate supervision than other social workers. Belkin-Martinez (2004) points out that the difficult and on-the-spot decisions that public child welfare workers must frequently make are often given intense media scrutiny. It has also been noted that evidently low support from administrators and supervisors is a leading cause of turnover among child welfare workers (Barak, Nissly, and Levin 2001; Rycraft 1994; Samantrai 1992; US Government Accounting Office 1995).

Role dilemmas

Liberation health practitioners who find themselves in the child welfare field face several dilemmas in their practice. These dilemmas can have a large impact on workers themselves, the way they relate to clients, and their ability to address dysfunction in their practice.

There is the dilemma of practicing social work, particularly from a liberation health perspective, with mandated clients. Involuntary treatment is often experienced by clients as oppressive and/or detrimental to their freedom (Ackerman, Colapinto, Scharf, Weinshel, and Winawer 1991; Adams 1992; Haley 1992; Weakland and Jordan 1990; Woody and Grinstead 1992). Naturally these factors may negatively impact client outcome (Glisson and Hemmelgarn 1998; Hemmelgarn, Glisson, and James 2006). Jennifer Sykes (2011) provides an important insight into clients' experience of mandated treatment from a child welfare worker. Through her interviews of women accused of child neglect, she noticed a recurring theme: mothers tend to consider themselves positively, resent the intervention of child welfare workers, and subsequently resist cooperating with service plans, even when it jeopardizes their custody of their children. From this, Sykes extrapolates:

> I find that though both CPS and mothers express a common interest in the wellbeing of the children, each group is enmeshed in separate dynamics (caseworkers needing culpability from mothers; mothers needing positive parental identity) which ultimately put mothers and caseworkers at cross-purposes.
>
> (Sykes 2011: Findings section, para. 4)

A social worker finding herself at cross-purposes with clients is unusual and ethically discouraged. As the NASW Code of Ethics (2008) notes in Article 1.01, "Social workers' primary responsibility is to promote the wellbeing of clients. In general, clients' interests are primary. However, social workers' responsibility to the larger society or specific legal obligations may on limited occasions supersede the loyalty owed clients." Mandated clients do not set the terms by which they are receiving services, nor the terms by which their services are terminated. As such, they do not choose what the goals of treatment are, and their interests are made secondary; specifically, their interests are superseded by the perceived interests of their children when they enter the child welfare system.

Of additional concern is the unequal treatment oppressed groups receive from the child welfare system. Families of color are overrepresented in the system and receive harsher treatment for the same behaviors (Roberts 2003). In this light, it can be difficult to say whether workers are tasked with protecting children or punishing mothers for being poor and of color (Appell 1996; Roberts 2003).

Lastly, a constant concern whenever clients' interests are not primary is that the interests of oppressive structures are being served. Throughout history, the interests of social and economic elites have been pursued in the guise of social welfare. If a caregiver is being asked to sacrifice, how are we to be sure that children are benefiting, and not oppressive structures? Liberation health practitioners are obligated to deconstruct mainstream ideological ideas of child welfare. Is the mainstream view of child welfare congruent with the cultural views and lived experiences of clients? Are these ideas eurocentric? Are they consumerist? Do they overemphasize individualism and ignore community, co-reliance, and collective responsibility? Child welfare workers represent state power in that they can break up families, and they may represent that state's interests by keeping families within the confines of the dominant culture's moral values and practices.

Case presentation

Presenting issue

At the time of the present case, Mary was a white, heterosexual social work student in her late 20s. She had worked as a public child welfare worker for several years prior to matriculating to graduate school in a major city nearby to earn her Masters in Social Work as part of a continuing education program at her agency. As part of the program, she was able to continue working at her agency on a part time basis for credit towards her degree.

As an exercise in experiential learning, Mary was expected to design and implement an agency level intervention as part of her curriculum. The first step in the project was to identify an "obstacle to service delivery." Mary, having a wealth of experience with her agency to draw upon, decided to focus on negative talk about clients among agency workers.

Over the course of her time as a public child welfare worker and then as a social work intern, Mary had noticed how frequently she and many of her co-workers "vented" about clients and their families in disrespectful terms. This venting ranged from expressing frustrations to derogatory or labeling language. Clients might be described as a "druggie," a "deadbeat dad," or even "my client the 'crack addicted mother'," among other things. Focus was particularly placed on recurring substance abuse or "resistance" to treatment. Occasionally she noticed an apparent lack of empathy, "Oh, this mother just doesn't get it! Why can't she understand why she lost her kids?" Other times workers could seem vindictive, commenting, for instance, that clients deserved having their families broken up by not complying with their worker's instructions.

Such occurrences were counter to Mary's own commitment to strengths-based social work and, indeed, that of many of her coworkers. In Mary's view, this negativity about clients was hindering service delivery, undermining therapeutic rapport, cultivating hopelessness in clients and workers, and creating a negative work environment for her and her colleagues. The literature suggests that she was correct; she was noticing signs of burnout and blaming the victim in herself and other workers at her agency.

Formulation

Mary began addressing this problem by attempting to formulate it using a liberation health lens. Accordingly, she considered this negative talk of clients from the three different perspectives suggested by Freire: personal, cultural, and institutional.

Personal perspective

Mary felt that she and her co-workers are likely to make occasional mistakes, or encounter obstacles they are not able to tackle in coordination with their clients, over the course of their practice. It is only natural that workers have difficulty reconciling this with their performance goals. In cases of missteps, many workers can be tempted to deal with failure by blaming it on clients instead of accepting personal responsibility. In other cases, individual intervention may not be sufficient in surmounting obstacles, and without having the tools to understand how failure may be caused by cultural and institutional forces, workers may default responsibility to their clients. Mary also noticed that many workers held onto lingering prejudices that skewed their understanding of clients' behaviors. These prejudices brought preconceived ideas about identity (such as class, race, gender, ethnicity) and how these characteristics relate to different behaviors (like drug use and parenting practices) to formulation and intervention planning. Lastly, Mary thought that, for many, conforming to a frequently negative office culture was psychologically and professionally safer than standing up to it. It requires a great deal of courage to push back against a negative workplace culture because very real consequences, a loss of camaraderie, inclusion, advancement, and trust, can be meted out by coworkers and superiors.

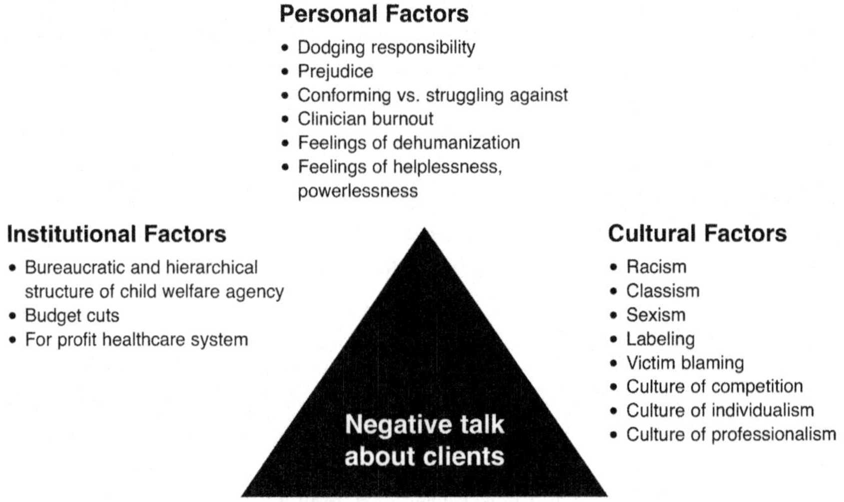

Personal Factors
- Dodging responsibility
- Prejudice
- Conforming vs. struggling against
- Clinician burnout
- Feelings of dehumanization
- Feelings of helplessness, powerlessness

Institutional Factors
- Bureaucratic and hierarchical structure of child welfare agency
- Budget cuts
- For profit healthcare system

Cultural Factors
- Racism
- Classism
- Sexism
- Labeling
- Victim blaming
- Culture of competition
- Culture of individualism
- Culture of professionalism

Negative talk about clients

FIGURE 9.1 Liberation health in a child protection agency
Source: Zack Osheroff

Mary also noticed other signs of burnout, in herself and in her colleagues, besides those related to depersonalization. She often found herself sleeping fitfully or not at all, particularly on Sunday nights, because she was worrying about clients and the many responsibilities that awaited her the next day. Among colleagues this was known as the "Sunday night blues." She also noticed people taking time away from the office because the emotional strain had become too much of a burden. Sometimes this took the form of a quiet walk out of the office. It also could be whole days off, known as "mental health days." These are all signs of emotional exhaustion. Negative self-evaluation was evident as well, as Mary knew many workers left the agency because they struggled with the power they exercised over others and yet did not feel they were creating positive change. This conflict invites negative self-evaluation, not just professionally, but morally as well. Mary herself often felt inadequate in dealing with the situations she was expected to manage, particularly when trying to build relationships with underserved and often troubled adolescents.

Cultural perspective

These personal factors influence, and are influenced by, many key cultural factors which also support the negative talk problem Mary identified. For example, the prejudices she noted in herself and her colleagues (many of whom are white and of middle class origins) are supported by dominant cultural messages that we receive about lower class people and people of color. It is therefore hardly surprising to find such messages shaping the perceptions of child welfare workers.

Additionally, Mary took note of the practice of labeling that is extensive in American culture in general and social work's culture in particular. Labeling is considered an effective way to communicate information about mental illness, disease, substance abuse, and a host of other problems that social workers and other helping professionals encounter in their work with clients. The American Psychological Association *Diagnostic and Statistical Manual of Mental Disorders*, the social science literature, guidelines developed by care management institutions, and often our own case notes, are all riddled with examples, and in fact may depend on using labels as a shorthand. This communication expedient has clear downsides. It is only natural that the same linguistic conventions that cause us to label someone struggling with schizophrenia as a "schizophrenic," would tempt us to use more detrimental labeling language for other behaviors, like drug addiction (a "crack addict") or child support delinquency (a "deadbeat dad"). This sort of language undermines the therapeutic alliance, making it easier to treat clients as objects. It also may cause us to see the source of problems as the clients themselves rather than the interaction between clients and their environment. This is a form of blaming the victim.

Mary noticed that the negative talk she overheard or participated in often construed the problems that clients faced as the fault of those clients. This victim blaming occurred because Mary and her co-workers received constant cultural messages that they ought to understand problems this way. She believed that client blaming often happened because the larger cultural and institutional factors that were contributing to the clients' problems were hidden from view. The child welfare workers had not been trained or supported in understanding their clients' problems more broadly, and thus workers' formulations and interventions overly emphasized individual responsibility. Because of this, it often seemed to workers that regardless of the interventions they made, their clients were simply failing to make necessary changes to avoid acute disruptions to their families.

Lastly, Mary noticed a culture of workplace competition that mirrored the dominant culture. We are often told that competition is responsible for human ingenuity, hard work, and success. We see competition celebrated all around us, from little league ball parks to reality television shows to the trading floor of the New York Stock Exchange. For these reasons, we often do not consider the negative consequences of approaching situations competitively. It may cause us to mistake potential allies, such as co-workers, for opponents. It can foster bitterness and resentment among community members. It can cause us to believe that one-upmanship is more important that empowerment, community, or solidarity. It can make us think that resource distribution or group interactions are zero-sum games. Mary believed this culture of competition was increasing the stakes at her workplace, making people feel the need to appear "more successful" to colleagues and supervisors. People were often vying to demonstrate who was willing to make the most sacrifices, who was most adept at getting clients to comply, or who had the most "expertise." This added considerable stress to the work environment and undermined mutual support and collaboration. It also reinforced individualistic ideas about work and success, prompting Mary and many colleagues to feel that they alone were responsible for their clients and that they could not or should not rely on coworkers for help. This increased stress, reinforced negative self-evaluation, prompted emotional exhaustion, and thus led to increased burnout.

Institutional perspective

Mary continued her Freirian analysis by identifying a number of institutional factors, both within her agency and without, that could be contributing to the negative talk about clients.

Mary's agency was heavily bureaucratic, even more so than other social work agencies. Above her was erected a very structured hierarchy, and her performance expectations were highly rigid. This left little room for her co-workers and her to use their skills creatively or to make important agency decisions, which, in turn, greatly undermined their autonomy. It also created a strict system of accountability that was often removed from client feedback and therefore seemingly arbitrary. To support this arbitrary system of accountability were endless deadlines, statistics, budgetary concerns, office meetings, progress notes, and quotas, more than there was ever enough time to complete, and all of which left Mary feeling as though helping her clients and doing her job were not aligned. All too often it seemed that the results of all this structure were client situations not improving, hours being wasted, and social workers getting blamed for the lack of progress. In other words, Mary and her co-workers were encountering high role conflict, role ambiguity, and role overload, which were leading to symptoms of burnout.

Meanwhile, budget cuts were reducing the availability of many of the services that clients like Mary's would have relied on in decades past, not just within her agency but within the public and non-profit sectors in general. These cuts in social services often left people, and the social workers that serve them, to fend for themselves. Mary found herself explaining why help was not available more often than she was able to deliver assistance. Being forced into this role of "gate-keeper" can be very disheartening for social workers, as it is often experienced by the social worker (and client) as a failure to help clients and achieve the agency's mission.

Lastly, social work training generally and the training provided by Mary's agency specifically often neglects to account for the importance of environment in client formulation and problem solving. Historically, social work attempts to account for environment in its understanding of human nature (consider, for instance, the impact of Bronfenbrenner's (1977) ecological model or the legacies of the settlement house movement). These influences are no doubt integral elements of the social work ethos. However, these elements remain largely theoretical in nature, as we often downplay or outright neglect environment when training social work practitioners to formulate clients' problems and to intervene (Specht and Courtney 1995). Our environmental understanding of human behavior continues not to be well operationalized, and therefore is difficult to apply to practice. When workers dwell solely in the realm of the personal, neglecting the institutional and cultural, we tend towards stigmatization and victim blaming. Other institutions, such as managed care, mass media, welfare agencies, advertising, our economic system, and mainstream politics, collude in reinforcing the idea that all problems have a personal basis. In this way, many of the institutions with which Mary and her colleagues interacted left them with few tools that could actually empower them to avoid blaming the victim.

Intervention

When viewed in its totality, the problem that Mary identified can seem overwhelming. Mary realized that she could not change all these factors by herself, and even if she received great support from colleagues and supervisors, a campaign to fix all these problems was far beyond the scope of her project. Understanding this, Mary still wanted to brainstorm an intervention that would touch upon the cultural and institutional, and not just the personal, antecedents to the problem. Ultimately, she decided that she could accomplish this by introducing Freirian analysis to her coworkers and supervisors as a way of understanding their clients and themselves.

Mary hoped that by introducing her coworkers to the liberation health lens, they would be better able to recognize the many ways that society was negatively affecting their clients. In turn, workers would be able to adjust their formulations to be less victim blaming, target their interventions in more effective directions, and practice with more empathy and less stigmatization. Acknowledging the many obstacles for clients, such as racism, classism, poor education, underfunded community services, insufficient employment opportunities, callous and disempowering public programs, underfunded public transit, discriminatory law enforcement, and many others, could be liberating for social workers who had no explanation for slow progress other than themselves or their clients. Additionally, by enlisting supervisors, Mary hoped that training, supervision, and agency policy could be affected, which would mean a more permanent and significant agency shift.

Additionally, Mary believed that she and her coworkers, their attention drawn to the problem and given the capacity to understand it beyond personal failing, would begin the process of breaking down the cultural and institutional factors that were affecting them directly, and had led them to burning out and blaming the victim. As suggested in the section on predictors of burnout, they could begin to create a culture of accountability around racism, classism, sexism, etc., that would prevent blaming the victim; they could find ways to build social support to reduce stress, break down competition, and celebrate achievements. A liberation health analysis would show workers that they were not solely responsible for the burnout and victim blaming that was affecting their practice and would indicate the proper targets for intervention.

Mary found support among staff and administrators, and got to work planning and organizing her intervention. She secured a space and the resources she needed, and organized a well-attended and enthusiastically received training. Mary was careful to acknowledge her own struggle with negative talk about clients, and proposed working together with co-workers to curb this trend in order to better serve clients. She facilitated an analysis of negative talk about clients using the Freirian triangle so that everyone could understand the ways in which institutions and culture were contributing. Mary was surprised by the enthusiasm she was met with. Her co-workers were able to identify most of the cultural and institutional factors that she had, it was part of their lived experience after all. There seemed to be a consensus that the problem Mary had set out to address was indeed a problem, and it was being exacerbated by the conditions in which they were working.

Next, Mary led the group in analyzing several clients' situations, again using the Freirian triangle method, so that all the participants would be able to perform this analysis on their own. She hoped that, beyond adding a new tool to her coworkers' arsenal, she would extend their capacity to better understand their clients and thus avoid falling into the trap of victim blaming.

Mary asked her co-workers to fill out surveys on what they thought of the training and the method. The feedback Mary received about her training was overwhelmingly positive; participants felt that she had given them new information to bring to their understanding of social work and how to connect with clients. They also committed to speak about their clients with respect and hold themselves accountable to the way they felt social work should be practiced. Unfortunately, many participants thought they would not be using the triangle as part of their typical social work practice, and cited barriers like time and supervisory support. Furthermore the many cultural and institutional challenges that had contributed to the problem in the first place, and contributes to many more, continue to this day.

Despite this, Mary noticed a distinct change in herself and her agency. The amount of negative talk decreased as workers felt a new sense of commitment to ethical principles that had drawn them to their work in the first place. The acknowledgement of what all the workers already knew, that they were working under immense pressure, scrutiny, and workload with limited personal accomplishment and autonomy, seemed to lift a burden which had dragged down morale for as long as Mary could remember. Mary could see a major success from her intervention, even though it was only the beginning.

Reflections

In truth, the reader would be far better served if the person telling this story were Mary herself. While her agency seems comfortable with constructive criticism and pressure to change from internal sources, many in the organization were concerned that Mary's story might bring unnecessary external criticism. Mary was explicitly warned that her career may be at risk if she contributed her story to this volume. This is why Mary's identity had been changed and the specifics of her workplace have been omitted. This should not obscure the truth: that the obstacles explored in this chapter are not limited to Mary's agency, or even public child welfare as a whole. The literature reflects the fact that burnout and victim blaming are profession-wide struggles, and their solutions require many social workers, and clients, united in their commitment to positive change.

Freire spoke of praxis: to see, to analyze, to act (Belkin-Martinez 2004). He believed that praxis was constant and cycling, and that systemic change and the development of critical consciousness required a return to evaluation after action. Mary's intervention did not radically change her agency, but it did have a palpable effect and continues to reverberate through her peers. It left her, and her co-workers, more empowered, although it could not create major changes in the institutional and cultural factors.

Guterman and Bargal (1996) point out that in our rush to empower clients, social workers have neglected to consider our own empowerment. Their evidence suggests that this is a mistake; empowered social workers are more effective social workers. Mary can attest to the fact that empowered workers are more respectful and understanding, and less likely to suffer from the symptoms of burnout. Engaging in praxis at our own agencies in solidarity with our co-workers, such as Mary has done, is a necessary ingredient to this empowerment. It can be extremely difficult.

Like our clients, we are surrounded by cultural and institutional factors that undermine our self-efficacy. Sometimes we are even threatened with severe consequences if we stand up to the cultural and institutional factors that negatively impact us. Alone, social workers' ability to create change is limited. Mary was disappointed that her efforts did not result in systemic change at her agency. She was also surprised that so few of her coworkers were prepared to continue using a Freirian analysis in their work. But this is the nature of creating change, both among our clients and among ourselves. It can be slow and halting. It takes persistence, cooperation, and time. Mary did not end negative talk about clients, but she brought attention to the problem and began a dialogue about solidarity and the conditions in which social work is practiced. To move forward, Mary will have to continue to bring attention to the factors which support problems in her practice, and others will have to join her as well.

In conclusion

Social workers face many obstacles to optimal service delivery. These obstacles do not simply make our work more difficult, but they can lead us down the path of burnout and can cause us to blame the victim (our clients). The benefit of liberation health is two-fold. First, it provides tools to social workers so that we can understand our clients and the problems they face more completely. In so doing, it can help us to avoid burning out and adopting a victim blaming mentality. Secondly, liberation health provides a model for understanding the dynamics that are acting on us, as social workers, and thus empowers us to engage in praxis to create positive change in our world.

References

Ackerman, F., Colapinto, J. A., Scharf, C. N., Weinshel, M., and Winawer, H. (1991) The involuntary client: Avoiding pretend therapy. *Family Systems Medicine*, 9: 261–6.
Adams, S. G. (1992) Family therapy and the legal system: One therapist's ideas and experiences. *Topics in Family Psychological Counseling*, 1 (2): 23–9.
Anderson, D. G. (2000) Coping strategies and burnout among veteran child protective workers. *Child Abuse and Neglect*, 24: 839–48.
Anderson, M. B. G. and Iwanicki, E. F. (1984) Teacher motivation and its relationship to burnout. *Educational Administration Quarterly*, 20 (2): 109–32.
Appell, A. R. (1996) Protecting children or punishing mothers: gender, race, and class in the child protection system [an essay]. *South Carolina Law Review*, 48 (577): 600–3.
Arches, J. L. (1997) Burnout and Social Action. *Journal of Progressive Human Services*, 8 (2): 51–62.
Åström, S., Nilsson, M., Norberg, A., and Winblad, B. (1990) Empathy, experience of burnout and attitudes towards demented patients among nursing staff in geriatric care. *Journal of Advanced Nursing*, 15: 1236–44.
Azar, S. T. (2000) Preventing burnout in professionals and paraprofessionals who work with child abuse and neglect cases: A cognitive behavioral approach to supervision. *Psychotherapy in Practice*, 56: 643–63.
Bakker, A. B., Demerouti, E., and Euwema, M. C. (2005) Job resources buffer the impact of job demands on burnout. *Journal of Occupational Health Psychology*, 10: 170–80.
Barak, M. E. M., Nissly, J. A., and Levin, A. (2001) Antecedents to retention and turnover among child welfare, social work, and other human service employees: What can we learn from past research? A review and meta-analysis. *Social Service Review*, 75 (4): 625–61.
Belkin-Martinez, D. (2004) Therapy for liberation: the Paulo Freire methodology. Available online at http://liberationhealth.org/documents/freiresummarysimmons.pdf (accessed October 4, 2013).

Boyas, J. and Wind, L. H. (2010) Employment-based social capital, job stress, and employee burnout: A public child welfare employee structural model. *Children and Youth Services Review*, 32: 380–8.

Bronfenbrenner, U. (1977) Toward an experimental ecology of human development. *American Psychologist*, 32 (7): 513–31.

Carver, C. S. and Scheier, M. F., and Weintraub, J. K. (1989) Assessing coping strategies: A theoretically based approach. *Journal of Personality and Social Psychology*, 56 (2): 267–83.

Cohen, P. (2010) "Culture of poverty" make a comeback. *New York Times*, October 19. Available online at www.nytimes.com/2010/10/18/us/18poverty.html?pagewanted=alland_r=0 (accessed October 6, 2013).

Conrad, D. and Keller-Guenther, Y. (2006) Compassion fatigue, burnout, and compassion satisfaction among Colorado child protection workers. *Child Abuse and Neglect*, 30: 1071–80.

Cordes, C. L. and Dougherty, T. W. (2008) A review and an integration of research on job burnout. *Academy of Management Review*, 18 (4): 621–56.

Demerouti, E., Bakker, A. B., Nachreiner, F., and Schaufeli, W.B. (2001) The job demands-resources model of burnout. *Journal of Applied Psychology*, 86: 499–512.

Derezotes, D. M., Poertner, J., and Testa, M. F. (2005) *Race Matters in Child Welfare: The Overrepresentation of African American Children in The System*. Washington, DC: Child Welfare League of America.

Diestel, S. and Schmidt, K.-H. (2010) Direct and interaction effects among the dimensions of the Maslach Burnout Inventory: Results from two German longitudinal samples. *International Journal of Stress Management*, 17 (2): 159–80.

Elliott, K. and Urquiza, A. (2006) Ethnicity, culture, and child maltreatment. *Journal of Social Issues*, 62 (4): 787–809.

Emener, W. G. (1979) Professional burnout: Rehabilitation's hidden handicap. *Journal of Rehabilitation*, 45 (1): 55–8.

Featherstone, B. (1999) Taking mothering seriously: The implications for child protection. *Child and Family Social Work*, 4 (1): 43–53.

Freudenberger, H. J. (1974) Staff burnout. *Journal of Social Issues*, 30: 159–65.

Gilliam, F. D. (1999) The "welfare queen" experiment: How viewers react to images of African-American mothers on welfare. *Nieman Reports*, 53 (2): 1–6.

Glass, D. C. and McKnight, J. D. (1996) Perceived control, depressive symptomatology, and professional burnout: A review of the evidence. *Psychology and Health*, 11: 23–48.

Glisson, C. and Hemmelgarn, A. (1998) The effects of organizational climate and interorganizational coordination on the quality and outcomes of children's service systems. *Child Abuse and Neglect*, 22 (5): 401–21.

Gorski, P. (2008) The myth of the "culture of poverty." *Educational Leadership*, 65 (7): 32–6.

Greenglass, E. R., Burke, R. J., and Ondrack, M. (1990) A gender-role perspective of coping and burnout . *Applied Psychology*, 39 (1): 5–27.

Guterman, N. B., and Bargal, D. (1996) Social workers' perceptions of their power and service outcomes. *Administration in Social Work*, 20 (3): 1–20.

Haley, J. (1992) Compulsory therapy for both client and therapist. *Topics in Family Psychological Counseling*, 1 (2): 1–7.

Hansung, K., and Stoner, M. (2008) Burnout and turnover intention among social workers: Effects of role stress, job autonomy and social support. *Administration in Social Work*, 32 (3): 5–25.

Hemmelgarn, A. L., Glisson, C., and James, L. R. (2006) Organizational culture and climate: Implications for services and interventions research. *Clinical Psychology: Science and Practice*, 13 (1): 73–89.

Hiscott, R. D. and Connop, P. J. (1989) Job stress and occupational burnout: Gender differences among mental health professionals. *Sociology and Social Research*, 74, 10–15.

Houkes, I., Janssen, P. P. M, de Jonge, J., and Bakker A. B. (2003) Specific determinants of intrinsic work motivation, emotional exhaustion and turnover intention: A multisample longitudinal study. *Journal of Occupational and Organizational Psychology*, 76: 427–45.

Hutchison, E. D. (1992) Child welfare as a woman's issue. *Families in Society: The Journal of Contemporary Human Relations*, CEU Article 19, February: 67–78.

Kim, H. (2011) Job conditions, unmet expectations, and burnout in public child welfare workers: How different from other social workers? *Children and Youth Services Review*, 33 (2): 358-67

Jackson, S. E., Turner, J. A., and Brief, A. P. (1987) Correlates of burnout among public service lawyers. *Journal of Occupational Behaviour*, 8: 339–49.

Johnson, S. P., Sullivan, C. M. (2008) How child protection workers support or further victimize battered mothers. *Affilia*, 23: 242–58.

Lamb, R. (1979) Staff burnout in work with long term patients. *Hospital and Community Psychiatry*, 30: 396–398.

Landsbergis, P. A. (1988) Occupational stress among health care workers: A test of the job demands-control model. *Journal of Organizational Behavior*, 9: 217–39.

Leiter, M. P. (1989) Conceptual implications of two models of burnout: A response to Golembiewski. *Group and Organization Studies*, 14: 15–22.

Leiter, M. P. and Maslach, C. (1988) The impact of interpersonal environment on burnout and organizational commitment. *Journal of Organizational Behavior*, 9 (4): 297–308.

Lizano, E. L. and Barak, M. E. M. (2012) Workplace demands and resources as antecedents of job burnout among public child welfare workers: A longitudinal study. *Children and Youth Services Review*, 34 (9): 1769–76.

Maiter, S., Palmer, S., and Manji, S. (2006) Strengthening social worker-client relationships in child protection services: Addressing power relationships and ruptured relationships. *Qualitative Social Work*, 5: 161–86.

Maslach, C. (1982) *Burnout: The Cost of Caring*. Englewood Cliffs, NJ: Prentice-Hall.

Maslach, C. and Jackson, S. E. (1981) The measurement of experienced burnout. *Journal of Occupational Behaviour*, 2: 99–113.

Maslach, C. and Jackson, S. E. (1985) The role of sex and family variables in burnout. *Sex Roles*, 12: 837–51.

Maslach, C. and Pines, A. (1977) The burn-out syndrome in the day care setting. *Child Care Quarterly*, 6 (2): 100–13.

Maslach, C., Schaufeli, W. B., and Leiter, M. P. (2001) Job burnout. *Annual Review of Psychology*, 52: 397–422.

McGee, R. A. (1989) Burnout and professional decision making: An analogue study. *Journal of Counseling Psychology*, 36 (3): 345–51.

NASW (2008) Code of Ethics of the National Association of Social Workers. Available online at www.socialworkers.org/pubs/code/code.asp (accessed October 6, 2013).

Norvell, N. K., Hills, H. A., and Murrin, M. R. (1993) Understanding stress in female and male law enforcement officers. *Psychology of Women Quarterly*, 17 (3): 289–301.

Peidmont, R. L. (1993) A longitudinal analysis of burnout in the health care setting: The role of personal dispositions. *Journal of Personality Assessment*, 61 (3): 457–73.

Posig, M. and Kickul, J. (2003) Extending our understanding of burnout: Test of an integrated model in nonservice occupations. *Journal of Occupational Health Psychology*, 8 (1): 3–19.

Pretty, G. M. H. (1992) Psychological environments and burnout: Gender considerations within the corporation. *Journal of Organizational Behavior*, 13 (7): 701–11.

Roberts, D. E. (2003) Child welfare and civil rights. *University of Illinois Law Review*, 171–82.

Roth, S. and Cohen, L. J. (1986) Approach, avoidance, and coping with stress. *American Psychologist*, 41 (7): 813–19.

Russell, D. W., Altmaier, E., and Van Velzen, D. (1987) Job-related stress, social support and burnout among classroom teachers. *Journal of Applied Psychology*, 72: 269–74.

Ryan, W. (1971) *Blaming the Victim*. New York: Pantheon Books.

Rycraft, J. (1994) The party isn't over: The agency role in the retention of public child welfare caseworkers. *Social Work*, 39 (1): 75–80.

Samantrai, K. (1992) Factors in the decision to leave: Retaining social workers with MSWs in public child welfare. *Social Work*, 37 (5): 454–8.

Schaufeli, W. B., Bakker, A. B., and Rhenen, W. V. (2009) How changes in job demands and resources predict burnout, work engagement, and sickness absenteeism. *Journal of Organizational Behavior*, 30: 893–917.

Schwab, R. L., and Iwanicki, E. F. (1982) Perceived role conflict, role ambiguity, and teacher burnout. *Educational Administration Quarterly*, 18 (1): 60–74.

Shirom, A. (1989) Burnout in work organizations. In Cooper, C. L., and Robertson, I. (eds), *International Review of Industrial and Organizational Psychology*. New York: Wiley, pp. 25–48.

Smedley, A. and Smedley, B. D. (2005) Race as biology is fiction, racism as a social problem is real: Anthropological and historical perspectives on the social construction of race. *American Psychologist*, 60 (1): 16–26.

Söderfeldt, M., Söderfeldt, B., and Warg, L.-E. (1995) Burnout in social work. *Social Work*, 40: 638–46.

Specht, H., and Courtney, M. E. (1995) *Unfaithful Angels: How Social Work has Abandoned its Mission*. New York: Free Press.

Stevens, G. B. and O'Neill, P. (1983) Expectation and burnout in the developmental disabilities field. *American Journal of Community Psychology*, 11 (6): 615–27.

Stevens, M. and Higgins, D. J. (2002) The influence of risk and protective factors on burnout experienced by those who work with maltreated children. *Child Abuse Review*, 11 (5): 313–31.

Sykes, J. (2011) Negotiating stigma: Understanding mothers' responses to accusations of child neglect. *Children and Youth Services Review*, 33 (3): 448–56.

Toppinen-Tanner, S., Ojajärvi, A., Väänänen A., Kalimo, R., and Jäppinen, P. (2005) Burnout as a predictor of medically certified sick-leave absences and their diagnosed causes. *Behavioral Medicine*, 31 (1): 18–32.

US Department of Labor, Office of Policy Planning and Research (1965) *The Negro Family: The Case for National Action*. Washington, DC: US Government Printing Office. Available online at www.dol.gov/oasam/programs/history/webid-meynihan.htm (accessed October 6, 2013).

US Government Accounting Office (1995) *Child Welfare: Complex Needs Strain Capacity to Provide Services*. Washington, DC: US Government Accounting Office.

US General Accounting Office (2003) *Child Welfare: HHS Could Play a Greater Role in Helping Child Welfare Agencies Recruit and Retain Staff (HHS)*. Washington, DC: US Government Accounting Office.

Van Yperen, N. W., Buunk, A. P., and Schaufeli, W. B. (1992) Communal orientation and the burnout syndrome among nurses. *Journal of Applied Social Psychology*, 22: 173–89.

Weakland, J. H. and Jordan, L. (1990) Working briefly with reluctant clients: Child protective services as an example. *Family Therapy Case Studies*, 5 (2): 51–68.

Woody, J. D. and Grinstead, N. (1992) Compulsory treatment for families: Issues of compliance. *Topics in Family Psychology and Counseling*, 1 (2): 39–50.

Zabel, R. H. and Zabel, M. K. (1982) Factors in burnout among teachers of exceptional children. *Exceptional Children*, 49 (3): 261–63.

Zell, M. C. (2006) Child welfare workers: Who they are and how they view the child welfare system. *Child Welfare*, 85 (1): 83–103.

Zellars, K. L., Perrewé, P. L., and Hochwarter, W. A. (2000) Burnout in health care: The role of the five factors of personality. *Journal of Applied Social Psychology*, 30 (8): 1570–98.

10

WORKING IN PUBLIC HOUSING

Anne Vinick with Carol Swenson

Introduction

The work described here occurs in an urban, public housing complex of about 2000 people. Residents must qualify as "low-income" to live in the complex where they pay 30 percent of their household income towards rent. Thus, wait-lists are usually years long. The Department of Resident Services is made up of a small number of staff who work with residents in different areas, including workforce development and education, youth development, health and mental health, and community engagement. Participation is free and voluntary, and staff works from a strengths-based, empowerment approach. Support, referrals and opportunities to connect with others through programs and special events are provided and valued. Regularly scheduled therapy is rarely an option, owing to the large numbers of people who reside in the complex and the lack of staff time.

One of the authors, AV, is the Director of Resident Services at the public housing complex discussed in this chapter, and the only social worker on staff. She worked with homeless families before receiving her masters in social work (MSW) and since has worked in public housing settings for almost 15 years. The second author, CCS, is a professor emerita at Simmons College, where she taught clinical practice and community-based practice in the MSW and doctoral programs. Her practice experience has been primarily in community mental health centers in urban settings.

Urban public housing has been portrayed in the dominant media as dirty, depressed, and dangerous. Public housing developments are typically located in neighborhoods with low median incomes, high rates of poverty, and disproportionate concentrations of minorities (Newman and Schnare 1997). In a climate of profit over people and few affordable housing options, public housing is in high demand; it is not uncommon to be on a public housing waiting list for five to seven

years. What public housing means to its residents is beyond an affordable, permanent place to live. For many families, public housing is the alternative to shelters
and overcrowded, unsafe living environments.

This chapter reflects the three main components of liberation health: popular
education, anti-oppressive practice, and liberation psychology. In addition, it draws
from the literature on community and public housing as an ecological site. A community issue within a public housing development illustrates some of the concepts
of this book.

Review of the literature

Popular education (Freire 1973) has been a galvanizing perspective for practitioners
in various disciplines, health, education, social work, to name a few, who are also
committed to social justice. These practitioners, who have been seeking to address
power structures that maintain poverty and oppression, have sought ways to transform professional practices in the service of liberation from unjust power structures
and internalized oppression. Freire taught that oppressed groups can be
transformed through conscientization, through developing critical awareness of
forces that contribute to their oppression, and through learning tools to press for
greater social justice for themselves and others like themselves.

Anti-oppressive practice refers to practice which is significantly oriented to
analyzing the conditions of oppression which are at the core of many problems that
bring people to health and mental health centers. It is a term that is more common
in England and Australia than in the United States (Dominelli 2003). In the United
States, the perspective has been more fragmented, and it has been common to refer
to anti-sexist, anti-racist, or other practices. However, all of these practices can share
a common analysis of power and its impact. The concept of intersectionality has
begun to be used to bring the disparate elements into a relationship (Crenshaw
1991). In addition, it allows for a more subtle analysis of the differences as well as
similarities between these different oppressions, and the multiple effects, for
example, of ageism, sexism, and racism.

Liberation psychology has a tradition reaching back at least as far as Franz Fanon
(1963), a psychiatrist and revolutionary. He wove a connection between individual
psychological problems and unjust social structures. His intervention strategies,
short of armed rebellion, were limited, however. More recently, liberation psychology has been adopted as a perspective within psychology in the United States and
Latin America (Martín-Baró 1994). This is where the Freirean pedagogy has
become so valuable: it is an approach that can "start small," with a few, or even a
single, individuals. Some practice applications follow.

One well-conceptualized practice approach integrating these elements is the
empowerment approach to social work (Lee 2004). While the language is not
explicitly that of liberation health, the framework draws from Freire, anti-oppressive practice, and liberation psychology. Lee applies her approach to work with
individuals, families, and groups, focusing on empowerment at the individual,

relational, and political levels. Her work is with people who are multiply oppressed, particularly the homeless.

The most fully developed example of liberation health practice is the cultural context model (Almeida, Dolan-Del Vecchio, and Parker 2008). This model has been developed in two contexts in New Jersey: the Institute for Family Services, and the Affinity Counseling Group. There, clients are invited for either individual or family initial sessions where they are introduced to the concept that individual and family problems are "created and maintained by societal power structures" (p. 7). They are also introduced to their social justice sponsors, volunteers who are further along in self-and social understanding, and prepared to help newcomers. In addition, the families are invited into an educational process to explore the operations of power and control, and their reciprocal: the processes of collective healing. As with other family-centered approaches to practice, family and individual sessions, for both adults and children are held, as appropriate. However, at the same time clients attend social education meetings where they build critical consciousness through discussions of movies, handouts, and other materials. They join men's and women's cultural circles as well, which consist of same-gender individuals who continue the process of analyzing cultural socialization and choosing alternative ways to think and act. Through this integrated program, families heal the issues that brought them to the center, develop life-long connections, become sponsors themselves, and reach out to the community.

While Almeida *et al.* (2008), develop community with the clients who seek their services, sometimes social workers have the unique opportunity to provide services to a whole ecological unit. Such is the case for social workers who work in public housing developments. The hiring organization may envision a relatively traditional role of amelioration (Prilleltensky 2008) of individual/family stress and dysfunction. Nonetheless, it is an ideal setting for a social worker committed to social justice who wishes to work from a liberation health perspective. Residents are already a defined geographic community and share common concerns and statuses, notably limited resources, including limited access to power.

At least since the late 1970s (Lee and Swenson 1978), social workers have conceptualized public housing projects as ecological units, with opportunities to work at the individual, family, group, and community levels. Liberation health brings to this conceptualization a consistent focus on power as a dominant force and a whole new array of skills and interventions.

For the purpose of this chapter, neighborhood is defined as the exclusive area of buildings and land that is managed by the company for whom Anne works. Community includes area beyond the perimeter of the public housing development, but does not go beyond the city limits.

Identifying information, referrals and presenting problem

Carmen is a 41-year-old, Latina, single mother of two children. She is currently in school full time and living in lower-income public housing in an urban area.

Carmen was referred to an on-site social worker by the assistant property manager after Carmen's 15-year-old daughter had been in a fight while waiting for the school bus a few days earlier. The event was videotaped and then posted on a social media website, where it was shared among many residents. The management office staff also learned about the event. Carmen was called in to meet with the assistant property manager who was concerned, after meeting with Carmen, about "the stress in her life."

Carmen and I met individually once a week for seven months. Where we met was flexible; in my office, her home, or somewhere else on the property where her children could have space close by to draw or do homework. I also saw Carmen and her children in social settings at least once a month on the property, at the community center or on the street. Both of Carmen's children began individual counseling at their community health center soon after Carmen and I began meeting.

Current situation

Carmen had been a resident of the housing community for six years prior to our meeting. She lived with her daughter, age 15 and son, age 6. When we met, she was in her last year of schooling for her bachelor's degree in criminal justice. At our first meeting, she was extremely upset and angry about the incident at the bus stop and especially that the "entire community was talking about the video." She expressed feeling embarrassed, helpless and scared about possible legal ramifications and retribution. Carmen knew a lot of people in the neighborhood. Residents, both children and adults, would often come to her for help with paperwork, translations from English to Spanish and general advice. Carmen believed that this event tarnished her reputation as always "having it together" and being a good mother. Carmen recognized that she had been under a great deal of stress recently and had no one with whom to talk about it. She attributed this stress to her stepfather's death, the recent diagnosis of her son with a serious hearing impairment, and then the fight. Carmen blamed herself: for the fight, for the fact that that she didn't recognize her son's impairment sooner, and that she didn't spend more time with her stepfather before he passed away.

Through the first few weeks of discussing her feelings of embarrassment, I learned that Carmen had experienced feeling deep shame long before these recent events, as she vividly retold some stories. When she was seven years old, having moved from the Dominican Republic to the United States, her teacher verbally assaulted her on a regular basis in front of the class. Her mother also had been abusive; Carmen was made to kneel on raw rice for long periods of time and was whipped with a belt. Carmen views these forms of punishment as cultural but also as very painful, physically and emotionally. Another example was a few years ago, after buying treats for neighborhood children, she recalled her humiliation when another resident asked, in front of a large group of children and adults, if she had just gotten her food stamps.

Carmen explained that her life has been filled with too many ups and downs and that often, as soon as she thinks that things are going well, something bad happens. She blames herself and the choices she has made. She also put a lot of emphasis on the facts that she was living in public housing, not working, and receiving food stamps. She believed that these facts defined her as a human being. As time passed in our work together, she was more readily able to acknowledge the successes in her life and connect her negative experiences and feelings of self-blame to cultural and institutional oppression.

Individual and family history

Carmen was born in the Dominican Republic and never knew her biological father. Soon after moving to the United States when Carmen was seven, her mother met her stepfather and had another child. Carmen describes growing up in a new city as very difficult. Her mother struggled to make ends meet, and Carmen did not feel like she was getting the emotional support she needed, especially with a new baby in the house. She could not speak English at first and struggled academically and socially. She described her mother as protective and strict during this time; she was only let out of the house to go to school. She struggled through school and eventually dropped out after her mother moved the family back to the Dominican Republic when she was in the 11th grade.

After moving around a lot on her own since she was 17 years old, Carmen moved back to the United States when she was 23 years old when she found a good job and moved into her first apartment. Soon after, her mother followed her back to the United States and found an apartment close to her daughter. Their relationship improved when Carmen's first child was born. Carmen was 25 years old, and her mother cared for her daughter while she worked. Nine years later her second child was born. At this time, she had plans to buy a home with her savings. But the father of her children stole all of her saving after asking to borrow US$10 with her debit card. She resigned from her job and applied to live in public housing.

Formulation

Personal factors that influenced Carmen include low self-esteem and feelings of shame. Emotional and social isolation and abuse as a child contribute to these feelings, as did her experiences as a single mother. Her choice of partner, her stepfather's death and her younger child's recent health diagnosis caused Carmen to question her ability to make appropriate decisions. Lastly, although her daughter was not seriously hurt in the fight, it was the final straw for Carmen. She was unable to see the positive steps she was making in her life, such as school and attending to her children's needs more fully; she was ready to give up on everything, as she had when her children's father stole her life savings.

The culture of individualism over solidarity tells us that it is wrong to rely on other people or government assistance for help. We live in a culture of productivity, and

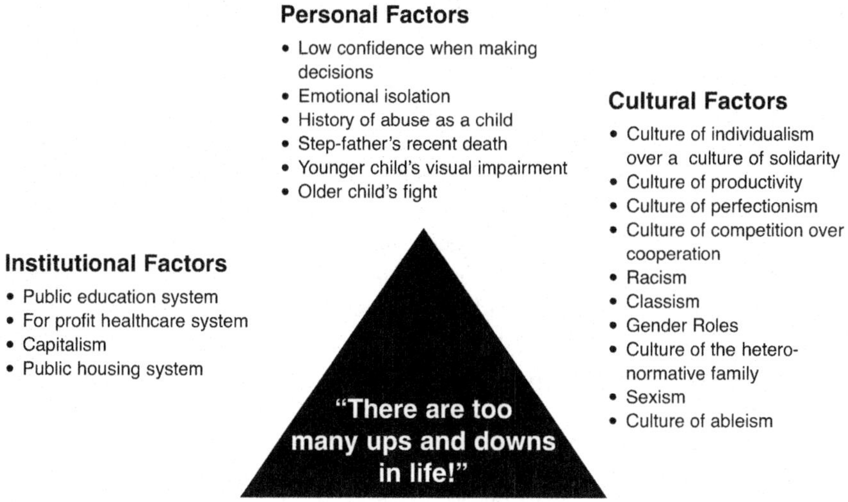

Personal Factors

- Low confidence when making decisions
- Emotional isolation
- History of abuse as a child
- Step-father's recent death
- Younger child's visual impairment
- Older child's fight

Cultural Factors

- Culture of individualism over a culture of solidarity
- Culture of productivity
- Culture of perfectionism
- Culture of competition over cooperation
- Racism
- Classism
- Gender Roles
- Culture of the hetero-normative family
- Sexism
- Culture of ableism

Institutional Factors

- Public education system
- For profit healthcare system
- Capitalism
- Public housing system

"There are too many ups and downs in life!"

FIGURE 10.1 Working in public housing

Source: Anne Vinick

Carmen sees living in subsidized housing and receiving food stamps as shameful and embarrassing. Our culture dictates that we are only as much as we produce and that only financial compensation proves our productivity. Our culture also places high value on financial success, and failure to achieve it is viewed as laziness and/or lack of intelligence. This dominant world view messaging constantly led Carmen to question whether she should be in school or be working full time. The culture of competition compels Carmen to constantly compare her life with that of other students in her classes and the people portrayed as "perfect" in the dominant social media.

Racism also greatly impacts Carmen's situation. In urban communities of color, violence and gangs are disproportionally prevalent; and the drug use, violence and crime that affect Carmen's family and so many others are not treated with the same seriousness as in white communities. Acts of violence occur every day, but only when they occur in white communities is it headline news. Carmen's daughter has been influenced by this cultural expectation, by law enforcement, the dominant media, and popular music, and it has negatively affected her and her family. Classism is also a cultural factor that contributes to Carmen's situation. Dominant culture tells Carmen that it is not important enough that she is a community leader and doing wonderful things in her neighborhood, taking care of her children and furthering her education; financial status is the bottom line. Colleges are organized for single, young people who have the luxury of going to school full-time, not caring for children and not working while taking classes. This is educational elitism that conforms to the needs of the rich and makes it more difficult for others to succeed and receive an equitable education.

Carmen's role as a woman and the corresponding responsibilities that she holds in and outside of the home are dictated by the dominant world view, which says that women are primary caregivers to children, cleaners and cooks. As a single mother, she not only feels responsible for all of these activities but also for the role that the dominant world view has traditionally dictated for men, worker, breadwinner, protector and disciplinarian. Carmen is torn between taking care of her children, her education and financially providing for her family. Sexism and the hetero-normative family of mother, father and children living together is relevant to Carmen's situation as well. As a single mother, and a person of color, she is stigmatized as sexually promiscuous or having done something wrong that created the family structure, which is seen by the dominant culture as less than desirable. Having a physical difference also clashes with the hetero-normative family. Carmen's son is now seen as "different" and needier by educators, classmates, healthcare professionals and society because of his hearing impairment. All of these cultural factors feed into not only Carmen's feelings of shame and self-worth but her children's as well.

In considering institutional and systemic factors, it is clear that the educational system failed Carmen from a young age. Overcrowded, crumbling urban schools with few resources and underpaid, frustrated and disinterested teachers are common problems associated with public education in many cities in the United States. These factors often result in high dropout rates; Carmen dropped out when she was 16. The healthcare system is also an institutional factor impacting Carmen's situation. Carmen took her son to the doctor for check-ups when she could, but the health clinic was understaffed and appointments were made months in advance. If Carmen missed an appointment, she had to wait months before her son could be seen. Doctors rush patients in and out, and the serious hearing impairment that Carmen's son suffers was not detected until recently. Carmen blames herself for not advocating harder even though she expressed her concerns for years.

Our capitalistic system prioritizes personal profit of the rich over basic human rights for all people. Although Carmen has worked hard, working or going to school full time and raising her children alone, she still struggles to feel worthy of basic human rights and happiness. The housing system reinforces this idea. Carmen dreams about moving away from the housing community where she lives even though she cares about it and her neighbors so much. Her building and apartment are in need of repairs, gangs and drug dealing lead to violence in the community, and residents do not feel like their concerns are addressed by management in a meaningful way. The housing system does not value her rights to a clean, safe place to live, rights which more affluent people may take for granted. It is no surprise that the people who are in charge of making decisions for the property are mostly White men who live outside of the city. Institutions and systems including healthcare, housing, capitalism and education along with cultural and personal factors, all significantly affect Carmen's feelings of shame and self-worth and attribute to the "ups and downs" in her life.

Intervention

It is our role as social workers to ask problem-posing questions to identify the cultural and institution factors, and raise consciousness about dominant world view messaging and how it relates to the problem. Carmen has many strengths, including her leadership in the community and her determination to complete her bachelor's degree while raising two children. In the liberation health model of seeing the problem through the eyes of the client, analyzing the problem together and acting upon the problem, it is also my role as clinician to help Carmen feel empowered to take action and support her goal to make change, moving from object to subject, in the context of the "ups and downs" that she describes.

Deconstructing the culture of individualism over solidarity was an important way for Carmen to feel less isolated and helpless. Individualism dictates the dominant world view that it is best to deal with problems alone, and that needing help is shameful. Carmen was taught that it was safer to stay away from people, that friends cannot be trusted and that she should not allow others to meddle in any of her personal matters. The culture of individualism was discussed after a few weeks of meetings with Carmen when she explained how difficult it was walking her son to school on time. Juggling both children in the morning was challenging. Her daughter took a bus to school, but since the fight Carmen waited with her at the bus stop. Her son had to walk, and there was not much time between when her daughter's bus came and when her son had to be at school. Walking to school in the morning was challenging, because of the large hills, extreme inclines and heavy traffic. Winter was treacherous as students were forced to walk in the street because of poor snow removal. Carmen didn't think it was fair that transportation was not provided. I asked Carmen if she thought other parents were experiencing the same difficulty. Carmen responded affirmatively, as many other neighborhood children accompanied her in the mornings, and parents learned to rely on her to escort them. However, Carmen had not spoken to other parents specifically about the danger of walking to school. She explained that it was not worth talking about it if there was nothing that could be done, and she feared being seen by neighbors as someone who complains. Together, we reframed this fear as a symptom of our individualistic culture. We thought about what it would be like if all of the parents got together to talk about school transportation and what it would feel like to know that others perhaps felt the same way she did. The idea of solidarity allowed Carmen to think about a different reality than the one she knew and question her own desire to stay silent.

As a person in an object role is manipulated and controlled by dominant, capitalistic systems, a subject influences and works towards individual and collective empowerment (Belkin-Martinez 2005). Talking to a few neighbors about school transportation was the beginning of a subject role. Carmen had been emotionally isolated for many years. Talking to a couple of neighbors about something important to her was a new experience. At our next meeting, Carmen excitedly told me about her encounters. Her neighbors did feel the same way that she did!

She explained how other parents had told her about their hardships getting their children to school, just like her. Their stories involved parents with physical limitations, those who worked nights and scenarios similar to Carmen's. The culture of productivity was highlighted at our next meeting. Carmen came in looking unenthusiastic. She explained that most of the parents that she knew were not working during school hours and that the school would think that parents were just being lazy for asking for a bus. It was important to raise Carmen's consciousness about the culture of productivity and how the dominant world view dictates that certain types of productivity are more valued than other types. Carmen later explained that many of these parents are working nights as cleaners or in factories and warehouses. Others had physical or mental health diagnoses that prevented them from working. We talked about certain types of work not being as valued as other 9:00–5:00 or higher-paying jobs. Carmen was conflicted as she spoke about her stepfather who had worked as a janitor his entire life. She admitted that she had always felt that it was beneath him, but now she was not sure why. I asked her whom she thought benefited from valuing certain jobs over others. She answered that the people in charge were benefiting, people who made a lot of money and White people.

Racism and classism were important factors to discuss with Carmen. As our discussion of school transportation continued, Carmen recognized that the decision-makers not only in the school system but also at the college she was attending were white professionals who had never experienced the hardships that she knew. I asked Carmen if she thought decisions would be made differently if school committee members' own children had to walk the same route. Were there different expectations for white children than for children of color, affluent children and poor children? It was clear that the people with power were not representing the students who attended the schools and their families. They had the money to own reliable cars and had choice about the neighborhoods where they lived. Yet they were making decisions, like the policy that transportation would not be provided to school if home was less than two miles away, by prioritizing "the bottom line" before the safety of children. Similarly, part-time status and evening classes were not available at the college Carmen attended. The decision makers at the college catered its class schedule, financial structure and lack of alternatives on the white, middle-class, hetero-normative family, a reflection of themselves.

Carmen gathered a group of six interested parents. The group decided to make a petition asking for a bus. Carmen was surprised by the passion of other parents around this issue. All parents would be asked to sign it, and the group could gauge interest and solidarity. Carmen and I continued to meet individually during this time. We discussed her amazement about how fast the issue was taking off and how people were really beginning to talk about this issue on the street, at the store, everywhere. She reported to me that her lack of energy was dissipating; she was more focused on her school work and was feeling generally more confident.

For three months mobilized residents had meetings at the elementary school, the school department and the neighborhood with the principal, assistant superintendent of schools, and transportation manager. A local non-profit got involved in the cause and advocated alongside them. After many passionate meetings and hard work, the assistant superintendent sent a letter to the residents informing them that a bus would be granted during the winter months solely for children of the housing development. He wrote that their argument behind the request was strong, and resident organizing efforts were impressive. Now, 80 children take the bus each day to school and back.

Reflection

As I reflect on my time getting to know Carmen and working together in the community, I often felt in conflict with my own white, middle-class background. This focused in three primary areas: my role as part of the management of the property while simultaneously aligning myself with residents, my privileged upbringing versus the oppression that residents of the property face and the fact that, although I have learned, I do not have the experience of being a resident.

Management vs. resident

As a colleague of the property management, I struggled with my responsibilities to uphold the rules and policies set forth by my employer, complete reports and produce a balanced budget while, at the same time, prioritizing my commitment to the goals and aspirations of residents. Since the early 1990s, resident service coordinators (RSCs) have become more prevalent in subsidized housing developments. Social workers and other human service workers understand the role of RSCs as advocating for and helping residents achieve their goals. The work of RSCs has been justified by property managers, asset developers and investors primarily due to the positive financial impact on the property; if residents are employed, financially and mentally stable, and have access to services, they are more likely to pay their rent on time and have less turnover of apartments. According to *Creating Opportunities for Families through Resident Services: A Practitioner's Manual* (Hyde 2006), resident services programs are best when they also support property performance. RSCs and management staff are thought by the department of housing and urban development to work as a team but this dual allegiance to both property management and residents has led to conflicts of interest and ethical dilemmas for RSCs. The concept of a "double bottom line" of both resident stability and property stability is complicated, and situations arise when one has to take precedence over the other. In my experience, the property prevails every time.

This practitioner's manual (Hyde 2006) stresses resident risk factors for personal problems; such as, "inadequate education, an underdeveloped understanding of sound financial practices and a job market that is demanding more and more skills," (p. xii) in addition to personal issues of domestic violence, substance abuse and crime. However, there is another way of understanding the role of RSCs; that is, in the context of the liberation health model.

As Carmen and I worked together around the transportation issue, I was feeling similarly to Carmen; as Carmen initially believed that residents would see her as a complainer or someone who is lazy, I believed that when management learned why residents were organizing that they would feel the same way about the residents. As Carmen began talking with residents, I began conversations with management. Like Carmen, I was pleasantly surprised with the response. Since then, I have been reflecting on how I was led to assume management's response and what messages I have been given as an employee. It will be important for me to provide them with feedback as residents are also inclined to have similar feelings.

Privileged vs. oppressed

As a white, middle-class woman working within systems that are dominated by white people, I felt a discomfort that I was taken more seriously and listened to more closely than the residents, none of whom were white. Because of my position, I was also seen as someone with power, and with access to people and information that residents did not normally have. When school representatives spoke, their eyes focused on me, as if I were the only one in the room. When asked a question, I would turn to community leaders to respond. Carmen, and other residents, were the experts.

Resident vs. non-resident

I felt privileged to be a part of this community organizing effort and that Carmen trusted me enough to share her journey with me. Carmen taught me a lot about what it was like to be a resident. We discussed that working in a community is vastly different from living in a community. Our differences were the basis for many of our discussions. Through praxis, to see, analyze and act, Carmen and I shared knowledge and a new understanding for not only the "ups and downs" in her life, but also how residents can successfully organize, and the positive impact organizing efforts can have on individuals and communities.

Conclusion

This chapter has shown the application of the liberation health model in the unique community of public housing. Though often viewed negatively by society, public housing offers an opportunity: a geographically defined area where residents share common experiences. Applying the concepts of liberation health allows the social worker to link individual distress to social conditions, and individual change to social action. As the client in the case example comes to understand how she has internalized the oppression she has experienced, she begins to see herself as someone who can mobilize other community residents and press for change at the institutional level of the school. The outcome is a more empowered individual, a more effective community, and the improved environmental conditions of a school bus for 80 children rather than a dangerous walk. The case example demonstrates how addressing individual disempowerment with liberation health analysis can lead to improved mental health, greater interpersonal competence, and greater social justice for a community.

References

Almeida, R., Dolan-DelVecchio, K., and Parker, L. (2008) *Transformative Family Therapy: Just Families in a Just Society*. New York: Alyn and Bacon.

Belkin Martinez, D. (2005) Mental health care after capitalism. *Radical Psychology Journal* 4 (2) Winter. Available online at www.radicalpsychology.org/vol4-2/Martinez4.html (accessed October 6, 2013).

Crenshaw, K. (1991) Mapping the margins: Intersectionality, identity politics, and violence against women of color. *Stanford Law Review*, 43 (6): 1241–99.

Dominelli, L. (2003) *Anti-oppressive Social Work Theory and Practice*. London: Palgrave Macmillan.

Fanon, F. (1963) *The Wretched of the Earth*. New York: Grove Press.

Freire, P. (1973) *Pedagogy of the Oppressed*. New York: Herder and Herder.

Hyde, C. (2006) *Creating Opportunities for Families Through Resident Services: A Practitioner's Manual*. Columbia, MD: Enterprise Community Partners.

Lee, J. (2004) *The Empowerment Approach to Social Work Practice*. New York: Columbia University Press.

Lee, J. and Swenson, C. (1978) Theory in action: A community social service agency. *Social Casework*, June; 359–70.

Martín-Baró, I. (1994) *Writings for a Liberation Psychology*. Cambridge, MA: Harvard University Press.

Newman, S. J. and Schnare, A. B. (1997) "… And a suitable living environment": The failure of housing programs to deliver on neighborhood quality. *Housing Policy Debate*, 8 (4): 703–41.

Prilleltensky, I. (2008) The role of power in wellness, oppression, and liberation: The promise of psychological validity. *Journal of Community Psychology*, 36 (2): 116–36.

11

LIBERATION HEALTH IN THE HOSPITAL

Dawn Belkin Martinez

Introduction

This chapter describes the use of liberation health theory and practice on a child and adolescent inpatient psychiatry service in a large urban hospital in the United States. The author, a self identified "liberation health social worker," worked in the hospital for 12 years and trained as a clinical social worker specializing in work with children and families. Following advanced postgraduate study in family therapy, the author went to Brazil to expand her knowledge base around Freirian models, popular education and liberation psychology. She came back to the United States and shared these new methods of practice with her fellow social workers at the hospital. Currently, she is a lecturer in the Clinical Practice Department at Boston University School of Social Work.

In many respects, liberation social work in a hospital may seem to be a paradox; hospitals tend to be somewhat hierarchical institutions and the medical model in general often employs an "expert" prescriptive lens/worldview around diagnosis and treatment (Belkin Martinez 2005; Williams, *et al.* 2005). As such, many of the liberation health practice methods utilized by this author and her social work colleagues were completely new to the inpatient service; doctors and nurses were initially skeptical as to how these interventions might be helpful to patients and their families. The medical team eventually was won over to support this conceptual framework and even institutionalized some liberation health language and techniques into their ongoing work with children and families. When interviewed for a local newsletter regarding the use of liberation health practice on the inpatient psychiatry service, the chief psychiatrist noted that he now considers this approach essential for patients to help them become active agents of change. He added that his team of social workers has had positive outcomes utilizing this model and that the work speaks for itself.

A brief review of the literature

Social work in a hospital

> It is because of the complexity of the social problems involved in the various groups of patients and the interdependence of the medical and social treatment, in any attempt at adequate solution, that the social worker is needed in our hospitals.
>
> (Cannon 1913: 34, as cited in Judd and Sheffield 2010)

Since 1905, social work services, beginning at Massachusetts General Hospital were an important component of patient care in hospitals (Judd and Sheffield 2010). "Doctor and social worker must each look to the other for the causes of the troubles he seeks to cure. At bottom, medical ills are largely social and social ills largely medical" (Cabot 1915: 105, as cited in Reich 2012).

Owing to the "person-in-environment" framework of our profession, social workers have been called upon to play increasingly important roles in executing patient care in US hospitals. Ida Cannon, one of the earliest hospital social workers, assisted Dr. Richard Cabot in developing a formal social work department at Massachusetts General Hospital at the beginning of the 20th century. As patient care began to include this additional practice component, social works' role in hospitals became increasingly prominent; by late 1930s there were over 1,600 hospitals that had formal social work departments (Judd and Sheffield 2010; Reisch 2012). During this same time period, social workers also became involved in providing psychiatric or mental health care. Influenced by the popularity of psychodynamic theories, hospitals began providing inpatient psychiatric services for patients, staffing many of these units with psychiatric social workers (Reisch 2012).

Today, social workers play key roles in administering care on many inpatient psychiatry units. Recent data from the National Center for Health Statistics indicates while the length of hospital stays among children and adolescents due to psychiatric diagnosis is decreasing, hospitalization rates for both children and adolescents have increased significantly (Blader 2011). Currently, it is estimated that almost 70 percent of total mental health costs can be attributed to inpatient psychiatric hospitalizations (Chung, Edgar-Smith, Baugher Palmer, Bartholomew, and Delambo 2008).

The adolescent experience on the inpatient psychiatry service

Adolescents who are hospitalized to inpatient psychiatric services do not fit a particular profile. They are diagnostically complex and present with a wide range of biological, social, and economic vulnerabilities (Cornsweet 1990). While the patients themselves come from different socioeconomic backgrounds, recent studies confirm that most adolescents admitted to inpatient psychiatry units are hospitalized for harm, or threats of harm, to self or others (Chung, *et al.* 2008;

Moses 2011; Romansky, Lyons, Lehner, and West 2003; Tonge, Hughes, Pullen, Beaufoy, and Gold 2008). In Tonge *et al.*'s (2008) descriptive study of adolescents admitted to a public psychiatric unit, he and his colleagues found that there were significant gender differences around the precipitating incidents facilitating hospitalization. Unsurprisingly, males presented with externalizing/disruptive behaviors while females exhibited more internalizing behaviors and incidents/threats of self-harm. Cornsweet (1990) found that families of patients were more likely to be socioeconomically disadvantaged, and another study found parent/child conflict to be related to more severe presentation and symptoms (King, Hovey, Brand, and Ghaziuddin 1997). Cornsweet (1990) also noted the hospitalized adolescents usually reported higher levels of family conflict than their parents.

Research findings on the factors which may predict rehospitalization for adolescents are inconclusive. Some studies report no relationship between psychiatric diagnosis/personality tests and readmission (Chung, *et al.* 2008; Romansky, *et al.* 2003) while others do find a correlation (Foster 1999). Several writers have pointed out that variables such as class, race, and gender have significant effects on mental health access, diagnosis, and treatment (Almgren and Lindhorst 2012; Reisch 2012; Star 1982; Wizmann and Anderson 2009). In their comprehensive study on health disparities, Braveman and colleagues (2011) point out that income distribution, housing, and a host of other environmental factors all affect access to and involvement in the mental health system of care.

Once hospitalized, many adolescents find the experience to be traumatizing and extremely stressful (Causey, McKay, Rosenthal, and Darnell 1998; Cohn 1994). They report feeling disempowered, disconnected, humiliated, and infantilized (Cohn 1994; Haynes, Eivors, and Crosseley 2011). In several qualitative studies of their subjective experiences, adolescents talk about the rigidity of unit regulations and hospital structures. They complain that their ideas about the program, and what might be helpful, are not taken into account and that many of the rules are both unnecessary and unreasonable. (Causey, *et al.* 1998; Haynes, *et al.* 2011; Moses 2011). The themes of disconnection, restriction/confinement and alienation were almost universally shared by all adolescents with one group of adolescents describing their inpatient experience as "living in an alternative reality" (Haynes, *et al.* 2011: 152). The loss of autonomy was also frequently noted; these feeling validate Abramsons' (1985, 1989) research in social work and ethics in which the social worker's experience of "doing good" is often more highly valued than client autonomy (Little 1992; Walsh, Farmer, Taylor, and Bentley 2003).

What's helpful

A review of the literature indicates that adolescents describe peer support and positive interpersonal relationships with staff and peers as the most helpful interventions during their hospitalization (Haynes, *et al.* 2011; Emond and Rasmussen, 2012; Kumar, Steer, and Gulab, 2010; Moses, 2011; Tonge *et al.* 2008). In her article entitled "Adolescents' Perspectives About Brief Psychiatric Hospitalizations: What is Helpful and What is Not," Tally Moses (2011) reported that, in her study of 80 adolescents hospitalized for the first time in a psychiatric program, most individuals experienced peer support as the most helpful component of their hospitalizations; the opportunity to receive feedback, mutual aid or solidarity, and normalization were noted to be "helpful ingredients of hospitalization" (p. 133). Similarly, Grossoehme and Gerbetz (2004) found that just being with other adolescents was reported to be the most meaningful aspect of inpatient care.

Interpersonal support and staff/treatment flexibility were also described as helpful interventions (Kumar, *et al.* 2010; Moses 2011; Tonge, *et al.* 2008). Positive inter-personal relationships with staff were tied to the adolescent's willingness to incorporate new coping skills, and their subjective experience of staff genuinely caring about them versus an individual just doing their job. Youth in Moses's study (2011) reported that they benefited from staff self-disclosure and appreciated staff's attempts to make connections and relate to them on a personal level. Most ado-lescents valued learning new skills, but again emphasized the human connection rather than specific techniques around skill development as most important to them.

Group therapy was also identified as a helpful intervention (Emond and Rasmussen 2012; Yalom and Leszez 2005; Yalom 1983). Finding common ground with others, validation from peers, and relief from isolation were all described as useful experiences of the inpatient group, and helped counter the effects of alienation noted above. Adolescents appreciated the "here and now" focus of the group modality and reported that the ability to make interpersonal connections and stay future-focused were more important than specific therapy techniques (Emond and Rasmussen 2012; Haynes, *et al.* 2011; Yalom and Leszez 2005).

Finally, several researchers identified parental support and involvement as a crucial component of successful inpatient treatment (Blader 2004; Brinkmeyer, Eyberg, Nguyen, and Adams 2004; Paterson, Bauer, McDonald, and McDermott 1997; Tonge, *et al.* 2008). As noted earlier, many adolescents report more problems in family functioning then do their parents (Tonge, *et al.* 2008), indicating the need to conceptualize treatment of the adolescents' psychiatric symptoms as just one piece of the total intervention plan. Paterson and his colleagues (1997) found that higher levels of parental involvement in an adolescent's inpatient stay were linked to lower readmission rates.

Liberation health and mental health treatment of adolescents

"Housing policy is health policy. Education is health policy. Neighborhood policy is health policy. Everything we can do to improve the quality of life for individuals in our society has an impact on their health" (Williams 2008, as cited in Reisch 2012: 889). While a review of the literature did not yield any formal studies of adolescent mental health treatment and the liberation health framework for practice, there were a number of texts and articles which linked mental health outcomes for youth and adults to sociopolitical factors (Braveman, *et al.* 2011; Lasch 1980; Timimi 2008, 2009). In their book, *Liberatory Psychiatry: Toward a New*

Psychiatry, Cohen and Timimi (2008) claim that the cultural values of consumerism, individualism and competition are significant factors influencing child and adolescent mental health. According to Timimi (2009) young people are socialized into a particular culture that teaches values, beliefs and practices that support the ideas of that particular culture at a particular moment in history. Mental health professionals often avoid analyzing how socio-political factors contribute to personal problems, focus exclusively on biological or personal factors, and take at face value that individual actions evolve from innate desires or personal dynamics.

Cohen and Timimi (2008) believe that our current super-narcissist value system, tied to the neoliberal free market ideology, decreases opportunities for support, cooperation, and solidarity, which in turn contribute to increasing levels of poor mental health for young people. The liberation health model, with its focus on a comprehensive socio-political analysis of personal problems and worldview deconstruction, may be an alternative method of practice which makes use of Cohen and Timimi's framework.

In their qualitative study of adolescents' experiences of psychiatric inpatient care, Haynes, *et al.* (2011) found that creating opportunities to chart new futures, tell new stories and experience new realities was a helpful intervention. These concepts are similar to liberation health practices of worldview deconstruction, introducing new information, and rescuing the historical memory of change. The following case example is an attempt to illustrate these practices on an adolescent inpatient service.

Case summary

Identifying information

This was the eighth psychiatric hospitalization for Sarah, a 16-year-old Anglo girl who lived with her parents and younger sister Tracy (13) in an upper-middle-class suburb in the United States. Her parents, Mr. and Mrs. Smith, had full custody of Sarah.

Referral and presenting problem

Sarah was referred to an inpatient psychiatric unit of a large urban hospital after cutting her wrists at school. For approximately one year she had been engaging in self-injurious behavior, including cutting her wrists, banging her head against a wall, and refusing to eat. The family had just been informed by the staff at her school that unless Sarah was able to "get these behaviors under control" she would not be permitted to return due to concerns about "Sarah's ability to be safe."

Course of service

Sarah met three times a week with her individual therapist, a psychiatry resident, and twice a week with her family and social worker for a period of two months.

Current situation

According to her parents, Sarah spent the last six months "bouncing in and out of the hospital". She was placed in a therapeutic day school seven months ago, after she was found cutting her wrist with a plastic knife in a bathroom of her public high school. Her parents noted that the-self injurious behavior "came out of nowhere," but that Sarah "never really liked school" and "seemed to have difficulty making friends." They had been hopeful that a new school would be a "fresh new start" for Sarah and were shocked that her wrist cutting and head banging incidents kept escalating, both in frequency and intensity. When asked by her parents and school providers what triggered these episodes, Sarah would shrug her head and say "I don't know ... they just come on ... I don't know why I do this and I can't control myself."

Upon admission to her new therapeutic school, Sarah began seeing an individual therapist once a week. Attempts to identify specific triggers to her self-injurious behavior were unsuccessful. After several months of therapy, Sarah was given the diagnosis of borderline personality disorder and prescribed a number of psychotropic medicines. Sarah hated her medication regime and reported she felt "drugged and out of it". One week prior to this hospitalization, Sarah was involved with a verbal altercation with her mother; she accused her mother of "trying to drug me" and flushed all of her medication down the toilet. Following daily incidents of self-injurious behavior, Sarah's mother brought her to the emergency room where she was assessed and transferred to the inpatient psychiatry ward.

At home, Sarah's behavior was described by her mother as "stressful ... she is stressing the entire family out and causing my husband and I to argue all of the time." Her father agreed and blamed Sarah for "wrecking the family." Initially, the family was unable to identify any of Sarah's strengths ... "she is just a train wreck". However, when asked later in the session, her parents talked about her kind personality and how wonderful she was with animals.

Individual and family history

Sarah grew up in a large home in an upper-middle-class neighborhood. Her mother was a full-time homemaker, and her father worked as a computer software consultant in Hong Kong. He "commuted" to Hong Kong, working continuously for ten days and then returned home for three to four days at a time. Sarah described her childhood as "OK, I guess"; she reported that her father had been commuting for almost ten years, and while she initially missed him quite a bit, now she was "used to it." Despite having "everything anyone could ever want" Sarah noted that her childhood was "lonely" and that she never "fit in" with the other girls in her neighborhood. When asked to elaborate more about not fitting in, Sarah recounted she had few friends as a child and that the "girls were into all those girl things ... you know dolls and stuff ... I wasn't." Sarah was an average student in school, but indicated that she did not enjoy her classes and mostly found her studies to be "boring."

Sarah was sexually abused by a babysitter for approximately two months when she was nine years old; she told her mother about the abuse following the last incident. The parents fired the babysitter and took Sarah for counseling at a local mental health center. Sarah went for counseling for several months and stopped going "because it was boring." Her mother reported the entire family went for counseling for several sessions, but her daughter seemed to be doing fine and the "counselor didn't see any reason for her to keep going." Sarah became very irritated when questioned about the abuse; "everyone keeps asking about this over and over again ... I barely remember what happened and it pisses me off that people keep bugging me about this." Again, she was unable to identify possible precipitants/stressors to her self-abusive behavior other than "being annoyed at people."

Sarah's mother had never received any mental health treatment, but acknowledged that she struggled with symptoms of both depression and anxiety. She reported feeling increasingly isolated and had days "when I don't feel like getting out of bed." Her mother described herself as an "anxious person" who frequently stayed up all night worrying. Sarah's father described himself as "normal, like my other daughter." He did not see his job as a possible stressor but did acknowledge that since Sarah "got sick" he and his wife were "fighting all of the time."

Formulation

Sarah is a 16-year-old Anglo female who presented to the inpatient psychiatry unit with a one-year history of self-abusive behavior and little insight into possible precipitants/stressors for this behavior. Sarah described her problem as a "ball of nerves affecting the entire family". In trying to understand all of the personal, cultural, and institutional factors influencing the "ball of nerves," a liberation health framework was employed (Belkin Martinez 2004).

Personal factors that may have affected Sarah include her history of sexual abuse, social isolation by peers, genetic predisposition to anxiety and depression, ongoing family conflict, and what Sarah characterized as her tendency to "bottle my feelings until I get really angry." She described herself as an extremely sensitive teenager who "bottled" perceived slights, and when she "couldn't take it anymore," would hurt herself. This physical pain distracted her from her internal distress.

There were a number of significant cultural factors and messages that contributed to the "ball of nerves". Most notable was Sarah's history of feeling left out with the other girls in her community and the messages to engage in gender normative behavior. Sarah spoke about the pressure to dress in particular clothing, engage in gender conforming activities, and behave in a prescribed "girly" manner. This feeling of "not fitting in" was longstanding and repeatedly manifested itself in her life, leading to feelings of alienation (I'm bored) and poor self-concept. Messages about gender appropriate behavior also affected both parents with Mr. Smith being locked into a narrow definition of what it means to be a man/provider and Mrs. Smith internalizing dominant world view messages about "how women

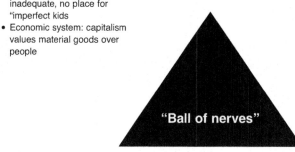

Personal Factors
- Social Isolation
- Rejection by schoolmates
- Low-self esteem
- Bottling
- Trauma history
- Genetic predisposition to anxiety
- Mother's depression

Institutional Factors
- Educational System-IEP inadequate, no place for "imperfect kids
- Economic system: capitalism values material goods over people

Cultural Factors
- Culture of individualism over solidarity
- Culture of consumerism
- Stigma
- Gender roles/sexism
- Culture of competition vs. cooperation

"Ball of nerves"

FIGURE 11.1 Liberation health in the hospital
Source: Dawn Belkin-Martinez

are supposed to behave." Sarah's mother also experienced feelings of isolation and disconnection, much of which could be attributed to the stigma attached to a mental health diagnosis and the culture of individualism. Moreover, the messages around the high value of consumer culture and competition influenced each family member and had a significant impact on the family's "ball of nerves."

The most prominent institutional factor contributing to the "ball of nerves" was Sarah's "one size fits all" school system. She was not a traditional learner and frequently felt like she was a failure at school. Additionally, the current economic system in the United States and Western Europe, capitalism, was ultimately also a factor which influenced the family's identified problem. While consumerism and competition are cultural messages that impact the ball of nerves, capitalism institutionalizes the prioritizing of the accumulation of wealth and profit over human relationships.

Finally, it is important to note that while the three categories of factors (personal, cultural, and institutional) are listed separately, they are not mutually exclusive categories; in real-life situations these factors interface and "drive" each other. For example, the cultural factors of individualism and competitiveness will influence the kinds of economic opportunities available and the educational systems that predominate. These systems further reinforce dominant worldview messages which then impact personal factors such as social isolation and poor self-concept. The process is recursive with all three categories of factors contributing to the "ball of nerves."

Practice interventions

Developing a shared vision of the problem

At the beginning of Sarah's hospitalization, identifying "the problem" and seeing it in its totality was a challenging task for everyone. When asked to describe the problems affecting the family, both parents initially reported that the problem was Sarah; if she would just stop this behavior, all "would be fine." Both Sarah and her sister disagreed with this assessment stating "it's not just Sarah … there is a lot of shit happening here".

The family was then asked to make a list of all of the problems affecting everyone, but was told that they were not allowed to put people on the list. In other words, they needed to think about what exactly was happening between people that lead to Sarah's hospitalization. Each family member developed her/his list of problems, and time was spent reading the lists aloud to the entire family and the treatment team. Common items on each list included "parents fighting all of the time," self abusive behavior, "not fitting in" and depression.

This writer validated their work and then asked the family if they would be willing to draw a picture of just one of the problems the family was experiencing. She acknowledged that while there were many problems the family was experiencing, the team needed to work with the family on one problem at a time. Everyone was encouraged to think about all of the different ways this problem affected individuals, the entire family, and the larger community.

After some initial bickering about which problem to chose, Sarah suddenly said "it's like I am walking around with a ball of nerves in my stomach constantly." Her mother and father quickly agreed with her assessment, noting that they too, felt as if they were walking about with a ball of nerves. Sarah and her family agreed that the "ball of nerves" would be the shared vision of the problem and drew a group picture, demonstrating how the problem of the "ball of nerves" affected everyone. This was an example of the Freirian method of developing a code to depict the group problem (Freire 2003).

Sarah drew herself a smiling young woman who had a large red ball in her stomach. Her father then drew himself frowning, with a red "ball of nerves" in front of his head. Mother drew a picture of herself in a car, driving to the hospital, with several red balls attacking the windshield. Sarah's sister initially stated she wasn't affected by the ball of nerves and drew herself as a stick figure in a bubble, listening to her iPad. Sarah challenged her sister, stating, "how can this not affect you … you said there is a lot of shit happening." Tracy reluctantly agreed and added a red ball into her individual bubble. Finally, the family shared their drawings with the hospital team members and indicated that while they still felt the process was "a little silly," it felt respectful and brought them together as a family. Sarah spoke at length about the fact that "nobody on the team called me a borderline" and that she liked that the language used with the family was "our language."

Analyzing the personal cultural and institutional factors affecting the problem

As noted repeatedly in other chapters of this book, a key component of the liberation health framework is the understanding that a family's personal problems are directly affected by ideology; that is, the dominant worldview messages individuals receive about the world and the institutions they interface with. In constructing the triangle of factors affecting the "ball of nerves," Sarah and her family were quickly able to identify the personal factors contributing to the identified problem. This is not unusual for families; most individuals are not accustomed to examining how cultural messages and institutions affect personal problems. However, the family initially found this writer's questions about socio-political factors affecting the ball of nerves "weird."

In attempting to meet the family "where they were at" and also expand the conversation, I asked Sarah to talk more about "not fitting in" with the other girls in her neighborhood. Sarah shared that, for as long as she could remember, she had felt "different from other girls"; she didn't like playing with dolls, dressing up and playing house, or "any sort of make believe or craft activities." As she got older, Sarah became more alienated from her peer group; she wasn't interested in clothes, boys, or, in her own words, "any normal girl activities." Parents acknowledged that Sarah was "different from other girls" and mother attributed this difference to Sarah being a "tomboy." This discussion led to my introducing the concept of dominant worldview messaging around gender roles; who decides what gender normative behavior is? Why are some behaviors by girls valued more than others? What would it be like for girls if all kinds of interests and behaviors were valued equally? Sarah, in particular, responded very positively to these discussions and eventually stated that dominant worldview messaging around gender roles was "f—ked up."

Once the family was able to expand the framework around the different factors influencing the ball of nerves, it became easier to identify other dominant worldview messages. Mrs. Smith talked about her own sadness and alienation and spoke at length about feeling left out of her large church community. She shared that members of her church often made food or ran errands for families that had children who were hospitalized or ill with chronic illness. Although her church community knew that Sarah was very ill and constantly in the hospital, fellow church members "look the other way if they see me coming and nobody has brought any food over to our home." When asked if she thought things would be different if Sarah had a physical illness, her mother responded "absolutely," and poignantly identified the stigma of mental illness as a significant contributing factor to her own stress level. Sarah's sister agreed and shared that if her sister was not around because of "cancer or something" her peers would be "nice and cool." Instead, Tracy developed elaborate stories about Sarah's whereabouts because of her shame about Sarah "being in and out of mental institutions."

This writer was very curious to learn more about Mr. Smith's job in Hong Kong and what that experience was like for everyone else. The entire family, including Mr. Smith, talked about how stressful it was to have a father gone "most of the time" and "just not available." This line of questioning led to another rich discussion about gender roles, consumerism and the culture of competition. The family discussed how important it was to have good cars, expensive clothing, and a well-furnished home. Sarah talked about the need to "have a lot of stuff" and joked about how, in her community, "you are what you own." Her father felt strongly that not only did he need to "provide" for the family, but he also needed to make sure they had "the same material goods as everyone else in the neigh- borhood." When asked if he thought having a job in Hong Kong and being gone for two weeks at a time contributed to the "ball of nerves" problem, he acknowledged it did, but said he "had to do it" because he was unable to find a job in the United States that "compensated me at the same level." Senior staff at Sarah's father's company were made aware of his daughter's frequent hospitalizations and overall problems at home. Yet, at no time during this year of crisis did company managers offer him a leave of absence or a reduced work schedule. Mr. Smith acknowledged that he never asked for any work accommodations "even when things were at their worst at home". He said that there is an unspoken rule at the company; "everyone knows you are there to produce … If you have any personal problems, you don't let them affect your work if you still want to be around."

This writer directly asked Sarah if she thought her experience with school (an institutional factor) affected the ball of nerves. As noted earlier, Sarah never really enjoyed school and usually described it as "boring." She identified herself as an experiential learner ("I like doing stuff, I don't like just sitting there and listening to the teacher drone on and on") and described school as painful since she was never a good student. Both Sarah and her mother were able to make the connect- ion between Sarah's own poor self-concept and the negative feedback she continually received about her school performance.

Taking action

Sarah's goal for hospitalization was simple: she wanted to get out of the hospital and stay out. When the family completed the action plan chart, everyone agreed that in order to stay out of the hospital, Sarah needed to develop positive coping strategies to utilize when stressed so as not to engage in self-abusive behavior. Their "long range vision" was to spend time together "outside of the hospital," and each member of the family identified individual activities they could undertake in order to help Sarah achieve her goal.

Sarah, together with her team, developed an affect management plan that focused on tiny "baby steps" to manage her anxiety. Along with a change in her medication regime, Sarah initially contracted to utilize positive coping techniques for just 30 minutes during the day. Some of the alternative behaviors identified by Sarah included putting ice on her arm when stressed, using her iPad in a quiet space, and playing with the unit's therapy dog. This plan was adjusted every few days until Sarah was able to spend an entire afternoon without hurting herself.

Setbacks were minimized; when they occurred, Sarah was encouraged to redirect her attention back to her goal (getting out of the hospital) and getting "back on the horse." Mrs. Smith agreed to stop threatening to send Sarah to a state hospital when her daughter had a "setback". Mr. Smith indicated he would call Sarah, his wife, and other daughter on a daily basis in order to "check in." Tracy stated she would stop teasing Sarah and say one nice comment to her each day.

Deconstructing dominant worldview messages, introducing new information, and rescuing the historical memory of change

While helping Sarah and her family to design narrative, cognitive, and behavioral interventions, I simultaneously engaged in liberation health practice by deconstructing dominant worldview messages, introducing new information and rescuing the historical memory of change (Belkin Martinez 2004). Following the identification of gender role messaging as a factor influencing the ball of nerves, Sarah and I deconstructed the messages our society puts forth on how women are supposed to look and behave. We read a number of feminist articles together and discussed who benefits when these messages are internalized. We talked about what it would be like if girls were not messaged constantly and what the world would be like if, in Sarah's words "everyone was just cool, that the way you were was fine … we wouldn't even have the term "gender nonconforming," because all ways to be a girl would be cool." We watched several videos about the women's movement and discussed the role of activism in changing not only legislation, but the way people think. This writer let Sarah know that when she herself was young, she couldn't even imagine a world where GLBT folks might marry. Sarah had no idea that activism had changed the public perception of gay marriage in such a short period of time. We talked about the dominant worldview message that things don't change, that you "can't fight city hall" or "the more things change, the more they stay the same." Rescuing the historical memory of change, through discussion of the victories of the women's movement, was very meaningful for Sarah and gave her hope that things could be different, that being "a different kind of girl" was just as valid and real as "being a girly girl."

We also spent quite a bit of time discussing dominant worldview messaging around gender roles for men and messaging around consumerism. As noted above, Mr. Smith felt strongly that it was his role to provide for the family. This writer asked Mr. Smith to elaborate as to what "providing" means and how the message of consumption, or in Sarah's words, "having a lot of stuff," might have influenced his perception of providing. This writer asked the family who benefits from this dominant worldview message regarding "providing."

Mr. Smith was initially annoyed by the question (what does this conversation have to do with Sarah cutting her wrists all of the time?). I worried that Mr. Smith might have felt blamed for working abroad. I validated his intention (wanting to "provide for the family), and at the same time raised the question around who benefits when this dominant worldview message is internalized. Both children indicated that corporations benefit from this message and stated that as much as they liked their stuff, they would prefer to have their father around more often. Mother acknowledged that she had also internalized this message and wondered what it might be like to think about "providing" in a different way. This paved the way for a discussion about alternative ways of living with "less stuff." The family watched a short video about consumption and read an article about families in Europe trying to live in a manner that deemphasized consumption and prioritized relationships and the environment. While Mrs. Smith and children were quite engaged around how consumerism/consumption were contributing factors to the ball of nerves, Mr. Smith remained skeptical, and I was always conscious of the need to externalize the message of consumerism so that he did not feel blamed. Interestingly enough, at Sarah's discharge meeting, Mrs. Smith shared with the team that her husband was in the process of looking for jobs within 90 minutes of their home.

Deconstructing dominant worldview messages about consumption facilitated a number of additional liberation health conversations. When Sarah's mother shared her feelings of isolation and sadness, this writer asked her if she ever felt that people were blaming her for Sarah's problems. Mrs. Smith immediately said she did, and acknowledged internalizing dominant worldview messaging around shame; that Sarah's problems were her fault and that if she had been a better mother, none of this would have happened.

This led to a discussion about the cultural value and messaging of individualism in the United States and again the question of who benefits when problems are conceptualized as private troubles as opposed to community issues. The entire family reported that they were not even aware that this was a message; that an individual's private trouble was their own personal trouble was "just the way it is." This writer referenced the article everyone had already read about European families and consumption and introduced an alternative message around solidarity. She shared her knowledge of examples of different countries that message a culture of solidarity and invited the family to imagine what that experience might be like for them. Mrs. Smith indicated that it would be wonderful not to feel blamed and shamed. Sarah suggested the family start rejecting the dominant worldview messaging around individualism and figure out "how to get more solidarity in our lives."

Finally, Sarah and I discussed her experience in a school system that values what Freire called the banking concept of education. In institutions applying this concept, students are passive objects that sit quietly while teachers deposit information into them. Students who have a learning style suited to this type of teaching are rewarded with good grades, while others are "punished" with bad grades. We introduced new information about the eight different types of intelligence (Gardner 1993) and Sarah enjoyed several videos about alternative schools which teach to many different learning styles.

The above action plan utilizes fairly common behavior management interventions, and the family work was consistent with basic family therapy techniques. What was unique about this work was the focus on deconstructing dominant worldview messaging, introducing new information, and rescuing the historical memory of change. To put it another way, we were making the direct linkage between private troubles/pain and public issues/problems. These interventions are not conceptualized as mutually exclusive from standard forms of practice, but rather an integral component of all assessments and treatment interventions. While this chapter presents the information in a somewhat linear manner, the reality is that the liberation health model is a way of thinking, a conceptual framework that can be utilized during any stage and time frame in direct practice.

Reflections

In many ways, the work with Sarah and her family was somewhat unusual for an inpatient service; she was hospitalized for almost two months and her parents came in for family sessions twice a week. Since she initially required so much attention, the treatment team spent a fair amount of time processing her ongoing situation and intervention plan. What follows is a summary of our reflections after the hospitalization.

The model was collaborative and Sarah and her family were in the "driver's seat" of developing her intervention plan. This observation is consistent with the literature concerning what adolescents find helpful about the inpatient experience. At times, it was not easy for staff to let go of their own preferences around action planning. I often felt frustrated with the (in my eyes) slow process around world-view deconstruction. On more than one occasion, I wanted the father to quickly challenge the capitalist/consumerist value system around the message to "have a lot of stuff" and instruct him to look for another job. Other staff wondered about the need for Sarah to "talk about her abuse history," even when Sarah clearly indicated she had no interest in doing so. A key piece of social work practice is valuing client autonomy and self determination, but, as noted in the literature review, respecting client self-determination on an inpatient unit is much easier said than done.

Analyzing the cultural and institutional factors that contributed to the problem positioned the team in a different relationship with Sarah and her family. During daily rounds, Sarah was initially referred to as a 16-year-old girl with a borderline personality disorder. Following identification of all of the factors contributing to her problem, the resident psychiatrist taking care of Sarah began presenting her in rounds as a 16-year-old girl with a ball of nerves that was interfering with her functioning. Understanding the multiplicity of factors affecting Sarah's behavior facilitated staff's treating her and the family in a different manner. This in turn facilitated the family's becoming increasingly engaged, with Mr. Smith flying in early to attend family sessions.

The literature identifies group work as a helpful intervention for adolescents on an inpatient service. I did not conduct any liberation health group sessions, but in hindsight, I believe that they would have been very beneficial for Sarah and the other patients on the service.

The liberation health model puts forth the position that the division between macro social work and clinical social work is a false divide; social work practice should include acting to challenge personal, cultural, and institutional factors that influence problems. There were times when I thought about asking Sarah if she was interested in attending a local march for woman's rights. However, given that Sarah's work in the hospital was focused on managing her self-injurious behavior, it seemed to be too much of a leap.

Two years after Sarah's discharge, I ran into her while walking downtown. I initially did not recognize Sarah, as she had cut her hair and was wearing "man tailored" clothing. Sarah was participating in a rally for animal rights. She seemed very happy to see her former social worker, but did not have much time to talk. I said a quick goodbye, picked up a spare sign, and joined the demonstration.

References

Abramson, M. (1989) Autonomy vs. paternalistic beneficence: Practice strategies. *Social Casework*, 70 (2): 101–5.

Abramson, M. (1985) The autonomy–paternalism dilemma in social work practice. *Social Casework*, 66 (7): 387–893.

Almgren, G. R. and Lindhorst, T. (2012) *The Safety-net Healthcare System: Health Care at the Margins*. New York: Springer.

Belkin-Martinez, D. (2004) Therapy for liberation: the Paulo Freire methodology. Available online at http://liberationhealth.org/documents/freiresummarysimmons.pdf (accessed October 6, 2013).

Blader, J. (2004) Symptom, family and service predictors of children's psychiatric rehospitalization within one year of discharge. *Journal of the American Academy of Child and Adolescent Psychiatry*, 43 (4): 440–51.

Blader, J. C. (2011) Acute inpatient care for psychiatric disorders in the United States, 1996 through 2007. *Archives of General Psychiatry*, 68 (12): 1276–83.

Braveman, P. A., Kumanyika, S., Fielding, J., LaVeist, T., Borell, L. N., Manderscheid, R., and Troutman, A. (2011) Health disparities and health equity: The issue is justice. *American Journal of Public Health*, 101 (S1): 149–56.

Brinkmeyer, M. Y., Eyberg, S. M., Nguyen, M. L., and Adams, R. W. (2004) Family engagement, consumer satisfaction, and treatment outcome in the new era of child and adolescent in-patient care. *Clinical Child Psychology and Psychiatry*, 9: 553–66.

Cabot, R. C. (1915) *Social Service and the Art of Healing*. New York: Moffat, Yard.

Cannon, I. M. (1913) *Social Work in Hospitals: A Contribution to Progressive Medicine*. New York: Russell Sage.

Causey, D. L., McKay, M., Rosenthal, C., and Darnell, C. (1998) Assessment of hospital related stress in children and adolescents admitted to a psychiatric inpatient unit. *Journal of Child and Adolescent Nursing*, 11: 135–45.

Chung, W., Edgar-Smith, S., Baugher Palmer, R., Bartholomew, E., and Delambo, D. (2008) Psychiatric rehospitalization of children and adolescents: Implications for social work. *Child and Adolescent Social Work Journal*, 25: 483–96.

Cohen, C. and Timimi, S. (eds) (2008) *Liberatory Psychiatry: Toward a New Psychiatry*. New York: Cambridge University Press.

Cohn, L. J. (1994) Psychiatric hospitalizations as an experience of trauma. *Archives of Psychiatric Nursing*, 8: 78–81.

Cornsweet, C. (1990) A review of research on hospital treatment of children and adolescents: A review of outcome studies. *Bulletin of the Menninger Clinic*, 54: 64–77.

Emond, S. and Rasmussen, B. (2012) The status of psychiatric inpatient group therapy: Past present, and future. *Social Work with Groups*, 35 (1): 68–91.

Foster, M. E. (1999) Do aftercare services reduce inpatient psychiatric admissions? *Health Services Research*, 34: 715–36.

Freire, P. (2003, 1970) *Pedagogy of the Oppressed*. New York: Continuum International.

Gardner, H. (1993) *Frames of Mind: The Theory of Multiple Intelligences*. New York: Basic Books.

Grossoehme, D. H. and Gerbetz, L. (2004) Adolescents perceptions of the meaningfulness of psychiatric hospitalizations. *Clinical Child Psychology and Psychiatry*, 9: 1345–59.

Haynes, C., Eivors, A., and Crosseley, J. (2011) "Living in an alternative reality": Adolescents' experiences of psychiatric inpatient care. *Child and Adolescent Mental Health*, 16 (3): 150–7.

Judd, R. G. and Sheffield, S. (2010) Hospital social work: Contemporary roles and professional activities. *Social Work in Health Care*, 49 (9): 856–71.

King, C. A. Hovey, J. D., Brand, E., and Ghaziuddin, N. (1997) Prediction of positive outcomes for adolescents psychiatric inpatients. *Journal of the American Academy of Child and Adolescent Psychiatry*, 36 (10): 1434–42.

Kumar, G., Steer, R., and Gulab, N. A. (2010) Profiles of personal resiliency in child and adolescent psychiatric patient. *Journal of Psychoeducational Assessment*, 28 (4): 315–25.

Lasch, C. (1980) *The Culture of Narcissism*. London: Norton/Abacus.

Little, M. A. (1992) Client self-determination: Current trends in social work practice. (Master's Thesis, California State University, 1992) *Master's Abstracts International*, 31 (01): 0155.

Moses, T. (2011) Adolesecents' perspectives about brief psychiatric hospitalization: What is helpful and what is not? *Psychiatric Quarterly*, 82: 121–37.

Paterson, R., Bauer, P. C., McDonald, C. A. and McDermott, B. (1997) A profile of children and adolescents in a psychiatric unit: Multidomain impairment and research implications. *Australian and New Zealand Journal of Psychiatry*, 31: 682–90.

Reisch, M. (2012) The challenges of healthcare reform for hospital social work in the United States. *Social Work in Health Care*, 51 (10): 873–93.

Romansky, J., Lyons, J., Lehner, R., and West, C. (2003) Factors related to psychiatric hospital readmission among children and adolescents in state custody. *Psychiatric Services*, 54 (3): 356–62.

Star, P. (1982) *The Social Transformation of American Medicine*. New York: Basic Books.

Timimi, S. (2009) The commercialization of children's mental health in the era of globalization. *International Journal of Mental Health*, 38 (3): 5–27.

Timimi, S. (2008) Children's mental health and the global market: An ecological analysis. In C. Cohen and S. Timimi (eds) , *Liberatory Psychiatry: Toward a New Psychiatry*. New York: Cambridge University Press, pp. 163–82.

Tonge, B. J., Hughes, G. C., Pullen, J. M., Beaufoy, J. and Gold, S. (2008) Comprehensive description of adolescents admitted to a public psychiatric inpatient unit and their families. *Australian and New Zealand Journal of Psychiatry*, 42: 627–35.

Walsh, J., Farmer, R., Taylor, M. F., and Bentley, K. J. (2003) Ethical dilemmas of practicing social workers around psychiatric medication: Results of a national study. *Social Work in Mental Health*, 1 (4): 91–105.

Williams, A. B., Burgess, J. D.; Danvers, K.; Malone, J.; Winfield, S. D., and Saunders, L. (2005) Kitchen table wisdom: A Freirian approach to medication adherence. *Journal of the Association of Nurses in AIDS Care*, 16 (1): 3–12.

Williams, D. (2008) *Place Matters*. Unnatural causes: Is Inequality Making Us Sick? Hour 3 [transcript]. Produced by California Newsreel with Vital Pictures. Presented by the National Minority Consortia. Available online at www.pbs.org/unnaturalcauses/hour_03.htm (accessed October 6, 2013).

Wizmann, T. M. and Anderson, K. M. (2009) *Focusing on Children's Health: Roundtable on Health Disparities*. Washington, DC: National Academies Press.

Yalom, I. D. (1983) Inpatient Group Psychotherapy. New York: Basic Books.

Yalom, I. D. and Leszcz, M. (2005) The Theory and Practice of Group Psychotherapy (5th edn.). New York: Basic Books.

12

WORKING WITH LATINO/AS

Estela Pérez Bustillo

Introduction

Latino/a or Hispanic is a term that is used to define a very diverse ethnic group. According to the 2010 Census, Hispanic origin can be viewed as the heritage, nationality group, lineage of the person's parents or ancestors before their arrival in the United States. People who identify their origin as Hispanic, Latino or Spanish may be of any race. The definition of Hispanic or Latino origin used in the 2010 Census is: "Hispanic or Latino" refers to a person of Cuban, Mexican, Puerto Rican, South or Central American, or other Spanish culture or origin regardless of race.

According to the 2010 Census, 308.7 million people resided in the United States on April 1, 2010, of which 50.5 million or 16 percent were of Hispanic or Latino origin. There has been a steady growth in this population over the past 40 years. It increased by 15.2 million between 2000 and 2010, accounting for over half of the 27.3 million increase in the total population of the United States. Population growth between 2000 and 2010 varied by Hispanic group. Among Central American Hispanics, those of Salvadoran origin were the largest group at 1.6 million (Ennis, Rios-Vargas, and Albert 2011).

The actual number of Latinos living in this country is even greater if we include in these figures those who did not participate in the census and the considerable number of undocumented Latinos who were not counted. One of the main characteristics of the Latino or Hispanic population is that it is predominantly made up of young members. Nearly half of the Latino immigrant population is under 25 years old and more than one-third is under 18 years old. One-fifth of the nation's children are growing up in immigrant homes and of these, more than 55 percent were born in Latin America (Pitman and Caro 2012).

Literature review

A liberation health model of working with Latinos is primarily based on the principles of liberation psychology. In the case of the large numbers of Latino migrants who are presenting with psychosocial issues in emergency departments or primary care practices in health centers or hospitals, providers need to be well versed in the profound impact of the US immigration system on their lives. The effects of immigration on the nation's economy and culture have been hotly debated over the past two decades, but the wellbeing of immigrant children has been largely ignored. The need for continuing research in the area of the psychosocial effects of the migration experience on children and families cannot be overstated. This section highlights critical concepts from several seminal works in this area of investigation.

Theories of acculturative stress

Migration entails a multi-faceted experience that implies adapting oneself to an unknown environment and at the same time experiencing the loss of family kinship ties, a familiar language and culture, and a system of social support. It often triggers various anxieties stemming from separation, stress, and persecution. Recent research on the process of immigration confirms that it is potentially severely stressful for immigrant children and families. Stress has been defined as "any event in which environmental demands, internal demands or both, tax or exceed the adaptive resources of the individual and environmental opportunities constrain the satisfaction of individual needs" (Menaghan 1983). Hovey and King (1996) define acculturative stress as the constellation of stresses, anxieties and shocks experienced by immigrants as they come into contact with a host society and change as a result of their interaction with it. In one of his studies, Hovey (2000) examined the relationship among acculturative stress, depression, and suicidal ideation in a sample of Mexican immigrants. Multiple regression analyses revealed that acculturative stress significantly predicted depression and suicidal ideation, while various other factors, such as family support, social support, agreement with the decision to migrate, and expectations for the future were mitigating factors. The findings highlight the importance of using culturally relevant clinical methods when assessing and treating the depressed and potentially suicidal acculturating individual.

The ecological-cultural-behavioral model of acculturative stress, developed by John W. Berry and his collaborators (Berry and Annis 1974; Pérez-Foster 2001; Hovey 2000), is the theoretical model that has been used by the majority of researchers working in this area. This model suggests that the extent and intensity of acculturative stress experienced by immigrants is a function of the characteristics of the individual and the group, as well as the relational features that are brought into the acculturation process by the immigrants themselves and the dominant society (Amason, Shrader, and Thompson 1999; Berry, Kim, Minde, and Mok 1987).

The school setting, where mainstream cultural norms and values are introduced and reinforced, is also the context in which the adaptation and acculturation processes occur. Some immigrant children experience considerable difficulty in adapting to the school system because they feel marginalized by their native-born peers, owing to the language barrier and their cultural differences. Child psychologists agree that being connected and accepted is an important component of adolescent development. Adolescents who do not establish meaningful connections with their family, their peers, or school are at an increased risk of suicide, substance abuse, school failure, health problems, and criminal activity. In some cases, the added stress of acculturation may exacerbate these risks. Adolescence, which is a particularly difficult time for most children, is especially challenging for immigrant children because they are trying to forge an identity in a "context that may be racially and culturally dissonant" (Garcia-Coll and Magnuson 1997).

Many studies on immigrant children have been carried out by educators. Carola and Marcelo Suárez-Orozco have spent more than 20 years working in the field with immigrant children. *Children of Immigration* (2001) is based on a research study known as the Harvard Immigration Project in which Carola and Marcelo Suárez-Orozco followed 400 children from five different countries or regions: Mexico, Haiti, China, the Dominican Republic, and Central America in a five-year longitudinal study. The book "is designed to provide an overview of the major themes in the lives of the children of immigrants – the nature of the journey to the United States, their earliest perceptions and their subsequent transformations" (p. 13). Chapter three is most relevant to this section because, in it, the authors examine the psychosocial effects of immigration on immigrant families and children, exploring the ways in which they deal with the gains as well as the losses, the opportunities and stresses of immigration on these families. The main stressors are traumatic border crossing, separation and reunification, violence in the new setting and adjusting to changes in family and gender roles. The authors also examine factors that contribute to the long-term adaptation of immigrants students, such as family cohesion, socioeconomic status, motivation for immigration, documentation, school quality and neighborhood safety.

Suárez-Ororzco, Todorava and Louie (2002) focus on the profound transformations that immigrant families undergo, which are complicated by extended periods of separation between loved ones, not only from the extended family members but also from the nuclear family. In cases where mothers initiate migrations, they leave their children in the care of extended family members such as grandparents, together with the father if he is still part of the family. When it is time for the children to arrive, sometimes they are brought into the country one at a time. Often, the reunification of the entire family can take many years, owing to financial constraints, as well as immigration laws. These migration separations disrupt attachments twice: first from the parent who leaves, and then from the caretaker to whom the child has become attached during the parent/child separation. The authors suggest that, in history taking, clinicians should always ask whether family separations have occurred. The psychosocial evaluation should include inquiries about patterns of migration, length of separation and the extent of family members' involvement. These separations are normative to the migratory process.

In their study on the impact of separation, Gindling and Poggio (2009) concluded that those who migrated at older ages (especially adolescents), undocumented immigrants and those who experienced a separation from their mother (compared to separation from their father) were more greatly affected. They are more likely to have strained relationships with parents and siblings from whom they have been separated. Gindling and Poggio's paper describes a successful program to ease transition to US schools for immigrants separated during migration. The model features individual counseling, group counseling sessions, and support groups that include peers who had also experienced family separation but who have been in the United States for a long time. Despite the fact that some school systems in the last several years have made efforts to improve English acquisition and educational outcomes among immigrant children, they have not created comprehensive programs such as this one to support these children as they undergo the usual stresses of childhood with the additional burden of major family and life transitions brought about as a result of immigration.

Liberation psychology

Liberation Psychology analyzes migratory phenomena in terms of power, and advocates for the transformation of societies at all levels (structural, organizational, and individual) as a means of promoting social justice and conditions of wellbeing for all social groups (García-Ramírez, de la Mata, Paloma, and Hernández-Plaza 2011; Paloma and Manzano-Arrondo 2011).

Oppression is a state of domination in which the dominant group obtains privileges over others by restricting their access to resources and limiting their capacity to respond. The immigrant population is negatively impacted by a variety of oppressive structural conditions which affect the immigrants' various spheres. These conditions have consequences on the collective level (feelings of alienation, passive attitudes), on the relational level (isolation, lack of participation) and on the personal level (self-esteem, depression) (Moane 2003; Prilleltensky 2008).

Liberation psychology developed in Latin America in the 1970s in an attempt to go beyond mainstream psychology. Its main exponent was Ignacio Martín-Baró, who suggested that this new way of doing psychology should have a social dimension (ending socioeconomic misery and political oppression) rather than focusing on individual liberation. It should also give priority to practical truth (have practical or social utility) over theoretical truth and have clear preference for the oppressed majorities. These principles are expressed by the author in this way:

> It is about putting psychological knowledge at the service of the construction of a society where the wellbeing of a few is not based on the lack of wellbeing of the majority, where the self-realization of some does not

require the negation of others, and where an interest for a minority does not demand the dehumanization of all.

(Martín-Baró 1985: 11)

The approach of liberation psychology denounces mainstream psychology as concentrating too much on the individual level and ignoring the structural causes and solutions to problems. It also promotes individual and structural liberation simultaneously, based on the conviction that both processes feed and depend on each other (Manzano-Arrondo 2011; Martín-Baró 1987). From the liberation psychology perspective, organizations play a key role in the promotion of a just, multicultural society. These organizations can promote social movements, recover the historical memory of the group in question, unmask the dominant narratives or the so-called "common sense" of the oppressor, promote critical thought and action amongst members of the community and campaign for the community's needs, struggling for its rights and denouncing injustice through political participation (Martín-Baró 1987). Brazilian educator and theorist Paulo Freire stressed the importance of creating a critical consciousness as well as the principle that knowledge for the sake of knowledge is useless. He believed that change will only occur when knowledge turns into action (Freire 2000).

Immigration advocacy

The immigration advocacy movement has strived to make the policymakers and legislators accountable for the oppressive nature of immigration laws and has fought for comprehensive immigration reform. Despite the fact that the mainstream media have adopted the word "illegal" to describe those who are not documented, it is only a federal misdemeanor to be in the United States without documents. For many years, immigrant rights activists have attempted to influence the public discourse to use the word "undocumented" and they have opposed using "illegal" as a noun rather than as an adjective to describe people's actions. One of the most eloquent slogans on placards in public marches supporting immigrants is the one that states unequivocally, "No human being is illegal!" The term "illegal" describes a social reality – inequality and lack of political and social status of a huge number of people who are forced into migration around the world. The impact of migration has been vividly demonstrated through the work of some journalists.

Photojournalist David Bacon has documented the relationship between labor, migration, and the global economy. Most contemporary migration is not optional but driven by globalization-related forces such as the demand for labor from industrialized nations. The exercise of state and corporate power reflects a worldwide trend in which global forces such as capitalism, patriarchy, and colonization continue to disenfranchise and dominate members of structurally marginalized groups, resulting in global problems of economic exploitation, poverty, war, terrorism, racism, and social exclusion. The first world's demand for service workers draws mothers from a variety of developing countries, often to care for "other people's children". In his book, *Illegal People,* Bacon (2008) exposes the human side of globalization, exploring how it uproots people in Latin America and Asia, driving them to migrate. Once they reach the United States, those who work without documents are viewed as breaking the law because of US immigration policy. Bacon summarizes this situation by saying, "A globalized political and economic system creates illegality by displacing people and then denying them rights and equality as they do what they have to do in order to survive – move to find work (Bacon 2008: iv).

The Pulitzer prize-winning book by Sonia Nazario, *Enrique's Journey* (2006) began as a series of stories for the *Los Angeles Times,* documenting the plight of unaccompanied minors who travel without documents from Central America into the United States. The main character of this non-fiction work is Enrique, a 16-year-old from Honduras, who makes the decision to travel alone to reunite with his mother, without telling her. He manages to elude the criminals who often prey upon these unaccompanied minors as they make their treacherous journey on the roofs of freight trains through Mexico until they reach the US border. Enrique's story proved to be an invaluable tool to engage the young man in the case study in a more objective analysis of the situation faced by thousands of minors like him.

Case presentation

Identifying information

Melvin is a 15-year-old young man from El Salvador who was referred to the mental health and social services department of a community health center to assist in his adjustment to reunification with his mother after an eight-year separation.

Referral and presenting problem

Martha is a 45-year-old mother of three from El Salvador, who requested an intake evaluation for her son, Melvin, who had arrived in Boston a few months earlier to join her and her second husband. Their reunion had been initially joyful, but they were undergoing a difficult adjustment to being a family with members who hardly knew each other, and who were living in a different culture than that of their country of origin. She described the stress she was experiencing at home between her role as wife and mother. Melvin demanded her constant attention, wanted displays of affection, and at times his inappropriate boundaries with her made her feel uncomfortable. He, in turn, seemed jealous of her intimacy with her husband and was competing with him for her affection.

Course of service

Martha sought assistance from her boss's wife, who was a resource specialist in the mental health department of the outpatient clinic where she received her primary care. It was the resource specialist's job to refer Martha to a bilingual/bicultural clinician for an intake evaluation. She asked me whether I had time to meet with Martha that day and introduced us. I met with Martha initially and then with Melvin. My work with them involved individual and family therapy and continued for about four months, as Melvin's behavior had improved by then and Martha had begun to see an individual therapist.

Current situation

At the time reflected in this chapter, Melvin had been living in the Boston area for a few months after being reunited with his mother following an eight-year separation. By this time, she was remarried and was living with her second husband, whom Melvin had never met. Martha worked as an administrative assistant to an accountant from El Salvador, and she had saved for several years in order to pay for a smuggler to accompany her son on his dangerous journey from El Salvador to the US border. Melvin was a reluctant therapy client, as he did not feel that he needed any psychological help, and he insisted that his mother was to blame for their difficulties.

Personal and family history

Martha's oldest son was Javier, then came Sara, and Melvin was the only product of her marriage to a man who was 20 years older than her, an army officer who died as a result of complications of diabetes when Melvin was four years old. After she became a widow, Martha struggled to support her three children on her own for a few years, until she made the difficult decision to leave her children with her mother and migrate to the United States in the hope of sending money home to support them. She had a friend who had settled in Boston and had promised to help her if she would join her there. When Melvin was seven years old, Martha left him and her two other children in the care of her mother in El Salvador and flew to Boston to start her new life. She was unable to visit them for several years because of her immigration status, but she spoke with them regularly on the phone and sent them packages with clothing, toys and school supplies. She also sent money to her mother to cover their expenses.

The only time Martha was given permission to return to El Salvador was when Javier committed suicide by hanging himself at the age of 20. According to Melvin, Javier used drugs and his girlfriend's father did not approve of him and had even threatened to kill him with a machete if he did not stay away from her. When she broke up with Javier and started seeing another young man, Javier was devastated. Melvin's grandmother found him hanging in the hallway outside his room in the middle of the night and she screamed, awakening Melvin, who also saw his brother hanging. He was only 12 years old at the time. Martha attended Javier's funeral and this was the first time Melvin had seen her in five years. His sister, Sara, was married. She and her husband had moved in with her grandmother, and they eventually had three children. Melvin wanted to go to the United States to be reunited with his mother, but he was sad to leave his grandmother and sister's family behind.

Formulation

Melvin's struggles with depressive symptoms and impulse control resulted from the intersectionality of his personal experiences and the social and institutional factors which helped to shape him (Freire 2000). Overwhelmed with the demands of adjusting to his new life in the United States, he chose to drop out of school and isolate himself at home. While this withdrawal was protective at first, it ultimately led to more social isolation and reinforced his feelings of inadequacy.

There were several other personal factors that affected Melvin, such as the loss of parental figures early in his life, namely, the death of his father when he was four years old and the separation from his mother when he was seven. His family had a trauma history highlighted by the tragic suicide of Melvin's older brother when Melvin was 12 years old. His maternal grandfather had also committed suicide many years earlier. The genetic loading for depression was present in three generations of their family. When Melvin was 15, he had to leave his grandmother, who was his primary caregiver, and his sister and her family, to make the journey from El Salvador to the US border accompanied only by a paid smuggler who could not be trusted, exposing him to the danger of being robbed, raped or killed along the way.

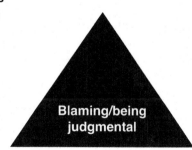

Personal Factors
- Genetic loading for depression
- Trauma history
- Grief/loss
- Intergenerational family conflict
- Social isolation

Institutional Factors
- U.S. immigration system
- Capitalism
- Educational system
- Child welfare system
- U.S. foreign policy

Cultural Factors
- Culture of militarism
- Dominant messages about gender roles
- Culture of machismo
- Stigma: "illegal"
- Racism
- Culture of individualism

Blaming/being judgmental

FIGURE 12.1 Working with Latino/as
Source: Estella Perez Bustillo

On a cultural level, Melvin had been socialized by his maternal grandmother in El Salvador into a fairly rigid system of gender roles which dictated that men must be self-reliant and strong in the face of adversity and never acknowledge that they need help. In part because of this attitude, Melvin was ashamed to admit that he was struggling to keep up with his academic work, so he did not get the help he needed in the first high school he attended in Boston. The culture of machismo, so prevalent in Latin American nations, dictated that violence is an acceptable way of dealing with conflict and this was also reflected in the threats Javier received from his girlfriend's father.

The culture of militarism was another value which had a strong influence on Melvin. His father had been an army officer and he was Melvin's principal male role model as a young child. It is no surprise that he aspired to a military career like his father. During the 1980s, the US-backed military had played a key role in El Salvador in fighting the civil war against left-wing guerrilla groups. US support also contributed to atrocities committed against the civil population of El Salvador, and his father had participated actively in this conflict. Melvin, as a 15-year-old young boy, was influenced by the messages he saw portrayed in the mass media to assert his male identity and enjoy the privileges it gave him. At times, Melvin reacted in an aggressive, impulsive manner in an effort to assert this male identity.

Melvin also felt the stigma of being an outsider, an "illegal", so vilified in current public discourse in this country. At times he would refer to himself as a "mojado" or "wetback", which reflects the degree to which he had internalized the negative stereotypes about undocumented immigrants that are so pervasive today. This internalized oppression was exacerbated by experiencing racial prejudice due to his brown skin and his facial features, which identified him as an ethnic minority. His self-esteem suffered as a result of these negative stereotypes and this exacerbated his depressive symptoms.

Melvin's situation is strongly impacted by several institutions, particularly the US immigration system and the capitalist economic system which fuels it. The forces of globalization displace workers from their homelands to other more industrialized countries where they are needed as cheap labor. This is one factor contributing to migration on a global level. Having entered the United States without documents, Melvin joins the approximately 11 million immigrants with undocumented status. He cannot apply for a driver's license, nor get a job like his American peers, because he does not have a social security number. There is no way for him to achieve legal status in this country under the present immigration laws. His mother cannot petition for him because she is not a permanent resident, but has what is known as temporary protective status. In the early 1990s, Congress granted Central Americans from El Salvador and Nicaragua temporary protective status as a result of the civil war in El Salvador and political instability in Nicaragua. There are legal initiatives which enable those immigrants "of good character" who could prove residency in the United States for seven consecutive years, whose deportation would result in personal hardship to remain in the United States to eventually apply for permanent residency and citizenship.

The educational system is another institution that has a huge impact on Melvin. In the Boston public school system, Melvin confronted the culture of individualism and competition, which made him feel marginalized. When he enrolled in the local public high school, he was placed in a class with students from many foreign countries, but they were expected to become proficient in English and function in the mainstream program within one year. They were not afforded the more gradual transition that bilingual education used to provide, nor was there a mentoring program available to assist them with their adaptation to the American school system. These barriers also interfered with Melvin's ability to relate to his peers, whose acceptance is so critical in adolescence. This alienation contributed to his social isolation, ultimately resulting in his dropping out of school.

Another institution impacting the life of Melvin and his family is the child welfare system, which became involved after his mother signed him out of the inpatient adolescent unit of a local hospital. His service plan involved outpatient therapy and a family stabilization team, which provided wrap around services for him and his family. The Department of Children and Families also paid for recreational activities which his family could not afford. Overall, their services proved to be an invaluable support for Melvin and his family.

It is clear that the combination of these personal, cultural and institutional factors contributed to Melvin's struggles and to his presenting problems. He was faced with the tasks of fitting into a new nuclear family with a mother he hardly knew and a step-father he had never met, navigating an unsupportive school system and finding his way in a dangerous urban landscape without speaking the language.

Interventions

Introducing the triangle

In meeting with Melvin alone for the first time, it struck me that he had very little understanding of the cultural and institutional factors which had influenced his mother's decision to migrate to the United States. He viewed it solely as a selfish, reprehensible act, and he was angry and resentful about what he viewed as her "abandonment of her children." Melvin tended to blame his mother and rarely looked at the external forces which had exerted pressure on her. In an effort to expand his worldview, I used the triangle and we spent a couple of sessions analyzing the cultural and institutional factors which influenced his presenting problem and situation. We deconstructed the socio-political conditions which made migration inevitable and Melvin realized that his mother ultimately had little choice in the matter.

Researching the problem

I decided to use Sonia Nazario's book as a tool to help Melvin learn more about the situation of mothers who have had to leave their children behind to migrate to the United States. I had the original book with colored photographs and maps, as well as the Spanish translation. This helped to increase his knowledge about the causes of migration and gave him a different perspective. The book also narrates the stories of unaccompanied minors who have made the treacherous journey over the border into the United States to be reunited with their mothers. Melvin was captivated by the photographs of these children and youth and their stories. We traced his journey from El Salvador, through Mexico, to the US border on the maps, and Melvin was able to see his situation reflected in a book that documents the experiences of young people like him. This allowed him to view himself as a subject whose situation is worthy of being documented, rather than as an object who is acted upon, or as a victim.

Developing critical consciousness

From the beginning of our interaction, it was clear to me that Melvin's behavior reflected traditional patriarchal values that he had learned in his extended family system in El Salvador, where he had been raised. In our individual work, we deconstructed Melvin's rather rigid, traditional male gender role identity and he was exposed to a more flexible model of gender identity. Deconstruction involved examining the account of his story and helping him to identify the implicit assumptions embedded in his narrative.

Melvin had come to Boston with the expectation that it was his mother's responsibility to take care of him and cater to his basic needs. He found himself living not only with her, but with a step-father whom he had never met. At first, he demanded a lot of attention from his mother. He was jealous of the affection she gave his step-father. He didn't like the fact that she and her husband sometimes took showers together. There was some inter-generational conflict because Melvin did not respect his mother's authority and he had a judgmental attitude towards her. In deconstructing his patriarchal values, Melvin began to see that gender roles are not as rigid here and that men are expected to help out at home and women often work outside the home.

Melvin reflected on his situation with his mother and realized that his expectation of being waited on was unrealistic within the context of their lifestyle in Boston. He developed more empathy towards her, which led to a shift in his behavior. He began to wash the dishes after she cooked a meal and eventually, with her guidance, he started to experiment with cooking, a skill he had never cultivated in El Salvador, where men were not allowed in his grandmother's kitchen. One day he arrived at the therapy session with a big smile on his face, beaming that he had surprised his mother by preparing dinner for the family when she came home from work.

Taking action

I realized that Melvin had very little grasp on his situation as an undocumented minor in this country when I heard his unrealistic personal goals after he dropped out of school. He planned to find a job but he did not understand that without a social security card and English fluency, this would be a huge challenge. I noticed that he referred to himself as an "illegal", but he needed to appreciate the dehumanizing aspect of that label and to find another term to identify with that was not so pejorative. We discussed the use of the term, "undocumented" as descriptive but not derogatory. Melvin became very interested in learning more about the history of US immigration policy, and he decided that instead of pursuing a military career like his father, he wanted to become an immigration attorney so that he could help the "undocumented".

In our discussions about his ambitions, I brought up the fact that he may not be able to attend college as a Massachusetts resident because of his immigration status. At the time, there was much controversy about the Dream Act, legislation being debated in Congress which would give legal status to youths who had been brought into this country without papers as children. Since these issues hit so close to home, Melvin was motivated to learn about the immigration reform movement. I told him about a group of activists who met in a local social service agency to advocate for changes in the immigration system, and he began to attend their meetings with a friend to learn more about immigration reform initiatives. These activities helped Melvin to identify with the community of undocumented migrants and to develop a sense of inclusion and solidarity. This activism also gave him hope that with pressure from grassroots movements, the US government might be compelled to initiate changes in its immigration policy.

At the time, Immigration and Customs Enforcement (ICE) was conducting raids in various communities in the outskirts of Boston. I was receiving phone calls from some of my clients telling me that they were afraid to leave their homes, and cancelling their appointments. There was an atmosphere of intimidation and fear within the immigrant communities. One day, someone from a local social service agency brought in a stack of flyers from an immigrant rights organization, which explained what immigrants should do if an ICE agent came to their door. The flyers were left in the staff mailroom at the mental health clinic. Later that day, the director of the clinic sent out an email stating that these flyers had no place in a mental health clinic. Luckily, I had seen them right after they were brought in and had taken a large number of them to my office. Each time I met with clients who were immigrants, I offered them the flyer if they wanted it. In my role as clinician, I, too, found myself moving from case to cause and from critical consciousness to action.

Reflections

One of the purposes of critical reflection is to challenge and change dominant power relations and structures, and to reconstruct possibilities for critical practice in contexts that are not necessarily conducive to this. As a clinician in a mental health clinic that relied on the medical model and was part of a large, urban teaching hospital, it was a challenge to integrate liberation health principles into my practice. I had to conform to the typical interventions and the demands of insurance companies to justify the medical necessity of the services that I was offering. I was fortunate to have a clinical supervisor who was very open to my ideas and wanted to learn more about the liberation health model.

In my interventions section, I focused exclusively on those interventions that were part of the liberation health model, but I also used other more traditional interventions. At one point, I had to act to protect Melvin when he became suicidal, facilitating his admission to an acute care hospital. I also filed a child abuse report with the child protection agency. These approaches reflect standard social work practice. Without a doubt, my way of working with Melvin and his mother was eclectic. If I have any regrets, it is that I only had a brief time to work with this family, since I saw them for only four months.

One of the factors that made it difficult to work with Melvin was the limited family and developmental history which was available to me. Since Martha had been separated from Melvin for a large part of his childhood, she only knew about the behavioral problems that her mother had shared with her. The behavior he was presenting could not be put into context with his earlier developmental history. The absence of this information forced me to focus more on the "here and now" and in retrospect, perhaps this was not a disadvantage.

When Martha disclosed to me in one of our monthly sessions that Melvin had threatened to take his own life by putting rat poison in his oatmeal, I helped to facilitate his inpatient hospitalization in an adolescent acute treatment unit. Melvin refused to take antidepressant medication and he begged Martha to take him home the next day, which she did. I felt that by taking him out of the hospital before he received a full evaluation and treatment for his depression, she was neglecting his mental health, so I filed a child abuse and neglect complaint with the Department of Children and Families, which was substantiated. At first, Martha felt betrayed by me, but when she saw the wide range of services provided by the Department, she realized that it was the best way to help her son.

The family became eligible for family stabilization services, an in-home counseling program provided by a team of bilingual/bicultural social workers from the Department of Children and Families, which proved to be very beneficial for them. The male youth worker who was part of the team exposed Melvin to recreational activities which he would never have been able to access otherwise. This young man also became a mentor to Melvin and was successful in connecting him to a basketball league in his community so that he could play his favorite sport. Without a doubt, this team effort of social supports and sponsors was a key element in Melvin's adaptation to his community.

Since I worked in a traditional mental health clinic, I had constraints placed on my time and my mobility, which limited my ability to make home visits or be more involved in the community. Another factor which limited my engagement with him as a youth was the age and gender difference between us, so the role of the youth worker was very significant in helping to bridge that gap. I realized that becoming a part of his community was one of the most important tasks for Melvin.

I wish that Melvin could have also participated in a group with other peers who had gone through the same migration and family separation. It is too bad that his high school did not offer such a program to help in the transition. A collective approach, which facilitates a process by which individuals name their experience and can identify with each other, can be very empowering. At the time I began to work with Melvin, he felt too ashamed to share his difficulties with his peers and he preferred to skip school to avoid confronting his insecurities. It was not until he transferred to a charter school that he found a mentor in the teacher's aide, who was also from El Salvador. He also discovered a peer group in that school, since many of the students had a similar background. He was allowed to take some elective courses there, and he particularly enjoyed a journalism course, in which he excelled because of his natural curiosity and writing ability. One of the first stories he covered was a May Day march of immigrants and immigrants' rights organizations that brought hundreds of protesters to City Hall. As the US Congress is poised to launch the first immigration reform legislation since 1996, it is my hope that Melvin will be one of the many who will benefit from the some of the changes being proposed.

References

Amason, A. C., Shrader, R. C. and Thompson, G. H. (1999) Newness and novelty: Relating top management team composition to new venture performance. *Journal of Business Venturing*, 21: 125–48.

Bacon, D. (2008) Illegal people: *How Globalization Creates Migration and Criminalizes Immigrants*. Boston: Beacon Press.

Berry, J. W. and Annis, R. C. (1974) Acculturative stress: The role of ecology, culture and differentiation. *Journal of Cross-Cultural Psychology*, 5 (4): 382–406.

Berry, J. W., Kim, U., Minde, T., and Mok, D. (1987) Comparative studies of acculturative stress. *International Migration Review*, 21: 491–511.

Ennis, S. R., Rios-Vargas, M., and Albert, N. G. (2011) The Hispanic Population: 2010. US Census Bureau. Available online at www.census.gov/prod/cen2010/briefs/c2010br-04.pdf (accessed October 6, 2013).

Freire, P. (2000) *Pedagogy of the Oppressed*. (30th Anniversary edn.). New York: Bloomsbury Academic.

Garcia-Coll, C. and Magnuson, K. (1997) The psychological experience of immigration. In A. Booth, A. Crouter and N. Landale (eds) , *Immigration and the Family. Research and Policy on US Immigration*. Mahwah, NJ: Lawrence Erbaum Associates.

García-Ramírez, M., De la Mata, M., Paloma, V. and Hernández-Plaza, S. (2001) A liberation psychology approach to acculturative integration of migrant populations. *American Journal of Community Psychology*, 47: 86–97.

Gindling, T. H., and Poggio, S. (2009) *Family Separation and the Educational Success of Immigrant Children*. UMBC Brief No. 7. Baltimore: University of Maryland.

Hovey, J. D. (2000) Acculturative stress, depression, and suicidal ideation in Mexican immigrants. *Hispanic Journal: Cultural Diversity and Ethnic Minority Psychology*, 6 (2): 134–51.

Hovey, J. D. and King, C. A. (1996) Acculturative stress, depression, and suicidal ideation among immigrant and second-generation latino adolescents. *Journal of the American Academy of Child and Adolescent Psychiatry*, 35: 1183–92.

Manzano-Arrondo, V. (2011) *La Universidad Comprometida*. Barcelona: Hipatia.

Martín-Baró, I. (1985) El papel del psicólogo en el context centroamericano. *Boletin de Psicológia de El Salvador*, 4 (17): 99–112.

Martín-Baró, I. (1987) El latino indolente of: Carácter ideológico del fatalismo latino-americano. In *Psicología Política Latinoamericana*. Caracas: Editorial Parapo, pp. 135–62.

Menaghan, E. G. (1983) Individual coping efforts: Moderators of the relationship between life stress and mental health outcomes. In H. B. Kaplan (ed.) *Psychological Stress: Trends in Theory and Research*. New York: Academic, pp. 157–91.

Moane, G. (2003) Bridging the personal and the political: Practices for a liberation psychology. *American Journal of Community Psychology*, 31 (1/2): 91–101.

Nazario, S. (2006) *Enrique's Journey: The Story of a Boy's Dangerous Odyssey to Reunite with his Mother*. New York: Random House.

Paloma, V. and Manzano-Arrondo, V. (2011) The role of organizations in liberation psychology: Applications to the study of migrations. *Psychological Intervention*, 20 (3): 309–18.

Pérez-Foster, R. (2007) When immigration is trauma: Guidelines for the individual and family clinician. *American Journal of Orthopsychiatry*, 71 (2): 153–70.

Pitman, K. and Caro, A. (2012) Immigration Experience of Latino Adolescents: Developmental Challenges. Paper presented at Adolescent Advocacy: Perspectives, Policy, Practice. Montclair State University, Montclair, New Jersey, 13 April. Available online at www.montclair.edu/media/montclairedu/chss/departments/childadvocacy/Immigration ExperiencesofLatinoAdolescents_Pitman.pdf (accessed October 6, 2013).

Prilleltensky, I. (2008) Migrant well-being is a multilevel, dynamic, value dependent phenomenon. *American Journal of Community Psychology*, 42: 359–64.

Suárez-Orozco, C., Suárez-Orozco, M. (2001) *Children of Immigration*. Cambridge: Harvard University Press.

Suárez-Orozco, C., Todarava, I. and Louie, J. (2002) Making up for lost time: The experience of separation and reunification among immigrant families. *Family Process*, 41 (Winter): 625–43.

INDEX

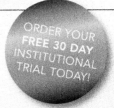

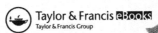

CPSIA information can be obtained at www.ICGtesting.com
Printed in the USA
BVOW09s1420081214

378199BV00004B/27/P

9 780415 698962